Understanding Self-Injury

Understanding Self-Injury

A Person-Centered Approach

STEPHEN P. LEWIS

AND

PENELOPE A. HASKING

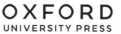

OXFORD
UNIVERSITY PRESS

Oxford University Press is a department of the University of Oxford. It furthers
the University's objective of excellence in research, scholarship, and education
by publishing worldwide. Oxford is a registered trade mark of Oxford University
Press in the UK and certain other countries.

Published in the United States of America by Oxford University Press
198 Madison Avenue, New York, NY 10016, United States of America.

Library of Congress Cataloging-in-Publication Data
Names: Lewis, Stephen P., author. | Hasking, Penelope A., author.
Title: Understanding self-injury : a person-centered approach /
Stephen P. Lewis, Penelope A. Hasking.
Description: New York, NY : Oxford University Press, [2023] |
Includes bibliographical references and index.
Identifiers: LCCN 2022044716 (print) | LCCN 2022044717 (ebook) |
ISBN 9780197545065 (paperback) | ISBN 9780197545089 (epub) |
ISBN 9780197545096 (ebook)
Subjects: LCSH: Self-mutilation. | Self-mutilation—Treatment. |
Parasuicide. | Parasuicide—Psychological aspects.
Classification: LCC RC552.S4 L49 2023 (print) | LCC RC552.S4 (ebook) |
DDC 616.85/82—dc23/eng/20221021
LC record available at https://lccn.loc.gov/2022044716
LC ebook record available at https://lccn.loc.gov/2022044717

DOI: 10.1093/med-psych/9780197545065.001.0001

9 8 7 6 5 4 3 2 1

Printed by Marquis, Canada

We dedicate this book to the countless people with lived experience whose resilience and generosity in sharing their stories has allowed us to write this book. Their silent strength is a constant reminder of the need to advocate for a person-centered approach in all aspects of research, clinical practice, and outreach.

CONTENTS

LIST OF ILLUSTRATIONS

FIGURES

BOXES

TABLES

Nonsuicidal self-injury (self-injury), the purposeful damaging of one's own body tissue (e.g., cutting) without suicidal intent, is a behavior that is a concern for countless people. Although it appears to run counter to the human instinct for survival—to avoid getting injured—self-injury can be the very way many individuals survive in the world. Often misunderstood, self-injury is primarily used to cope with intense or unwanted emotions that an individual feels they are not able to deal with in other ways. Not surprisingly then, self-injury is associated with a number of mental health difficulties (e.g., emotion dysregulation, major depression) and is a reliable predictor of subsequent suicidal thoughts and behavior. For these reasons there has been increased attention paid to factors that initiate and maintain self-injury, and a recent focus on factors that might aid recovery.

Over the past two decades, our understanding of self-injury has expanded significantly. Yet, self-injury remains shrouded in much stigma which foments shame, isolation, and hopelessness for countless individuals who self-injure. Accordingly, how we talk about self-injury and respond to individuals who self-injure necessitate an empowering approach conducive to fostering strength, hope, and resilience. In keeping with the recent strengths-based movements toward conceptualizing and addressing mental health difficulties, this book offers a novel person-centered and strengths-based framing of self-injury. In doing so, the book addresses contemporary and often overlooked areas in the field, such as stigma, recovery, and the role of social media in self-injury. Given its applied emphasis, this book will be relevant and useful to anyone working with or supporting people with lived self-injury experience, including: mental health professionals and trainees, school professionals, families, and researchers. We hope people with lived experience of self-injury find this book empowering, and consider sharing it with loved ones.

In the first part of the book we aim to contextualize self-injury. In Chapter 1, we start by outlining the most up-to-date understanding of what self-injury is, how common it is, factors that are associated with self-injury, and the relationship between self-injury and suicidal thoughts and behaviors. In Chapter 2, we further delineate self-injury from suicidal behavior, highlighting the similarities and differences between them, and proposing a person-centered way to inquire about suicidal thinking. We then move on to offering a person-centered framing of self-injury. In Chapter 3, we argue that many models of self-injury adopt a medicalized viewpoint—seeing self-injury as a symptom that needs to be treated and removed. These models frame self-injury as a problem that needs to be fixed, that arises due to some deficit or flaw in the individual (e.g., a history of trauma, lack of coping skills). We argue that a deficit-based approach can, perhaps inadvertently, emphasize vulnerabilities and feelings of worthlessness often held by people who self-injure. We offer readers a strengths-based approach that instead highlights the resilience of people who self-injure. While not dismissing factors that drive self-injury, additionally focusing on strengths can further empower people toward positive change and recovery.

Self-injury remains a highly stigmatized behavior, yet there has been little consideration in the literature regarding how stigma manifests, and the impact this stigma has on people who self-injure. In Chapter 4, we tackle stigma head-on, challenging readers to adopt a nonstigmatizing framing of self-injury. Along similar lines, Chapter 5 draws on recent work highlighting the importance of the language we use when talking about self-injury, and people who self-injure. Language is a powerful form of communication that helps frame the way we see the world. Stigmatizing, medicalized, or derogatory language—often used unintentionally—can foster shame and reduce the likelihood a person who self-injures will reach out for support. We present readers a guide on appropriate ways to talk about self-injury that foster respect, hope, and resilience. In this way, we hope people who wish to talk about their self-injury are able to receive nonjudgmental, noncritical responses to their disclosures.

In Chapter 6, we address the issue of self-injury "contagion." We present the latest evidence regarding social causes and consequences of self-injury among peer groups. Following our discussion of appropriate language to use when talking about self-injury, we consider the pitfalls of adopting a medicalized conceptualization of the social causes and consequences of self-injury, which is grounded in an infectious diseases model. Instead, we focus on how we can encourage a broader discussion of these social influences and effects associated with self-injury. This includes consideration of societal attitudes, discussion of self-injury in a broader social context, and response to people who self-injure. In Chapter 7 we broaden this discussion to social media. Indeed, there has been much concern about the effect of social media on self-injury, with many suggesting that online communication about self-injury can encourage people to engage in the behavior. Yet, others propose that discussing self-injury online can decrease isolation, and assist with recovery. We rely on recent evidence to present both the benefits and risks associated with online communication of self-injury.

The remainder of this book is focused on applying this person-centered approach across a range of contexts. In Chapter 8 we turn our attention to the roles schools can play in the prevention and early intervention of self-injury. Given self-injury most often emerges in adolescence, schools have become a prime context in which to identify students who self-injure and offer appropriate and timely referral. Yet school staff tell us they are unsure how to respond to self-injury, and are worried about "contagion" if they discuss self-injury with students. In this chapter we offer guidance for schools in adopting a whole-of-school approach and developing a policy to address and respond to self-injury. Acknowledging that all school staff have a role to play in appropriately addressing and responding to self-injury is important in developing effective school protocols. Extending considerations about caring for people who self-injure, in Chapter 9 we focus on how families can adopt a strengths-based approach in responding to a family member who self-injures. This includes the role of siblings, and consideration of how self-injury can impact family functioning.

Next we shift our attention to the recovery process. We begin Chapter 10 by taking a look at existing treatments for self-injury and critically appraise the evidence for their use. Against this tradition, there has been a recent move to direct attention away from factors that initiate and maintain self-injury to factors that help promote recovery. Traditionally, the focus of recovery has been on stopping self-injury. However, in Chapter 11, we propose a new way to conceptualize recovery that takes into account not just the behavioral aspect of self-injury but also associated beliefs and expectations about recovery. Building on the person-centered approach, we argue that recovery is an ongoing, nonlinear, individual process. This process is not just about finding alternatives to self-injury but also involves an understanding that setbacks can be expected, that thoughts and urges to self-injure can be ongoing, that scarring and disclosure of self-injury to others can be challenging, and that self-acceptance and self-compassion are possible. Building on this in Chapter 12, we apply this person-centered model of recovery to how people who self-injure can build resilience.

In Chapter 13 we begin by considering how to support individuals who self-injure. Although many resources are available to help people initiate conversations about self-injury, we acknowledge that supporting someone who self-injures is an ongoing conversation—and one that will change over time. In addition to providing guidance for parents, friends, teachers, and others who care for someone who self-injures, we offer people who self-injure a way to internalize the strengths-based approach in their own interactions with others. This includes considerations regarding disclosures, how to respond to questions about scarring, and the importance of self-care. Finally, in Chapter 14 we emphasize the need for advocacy of the person-centered approach through research, clinical practice, and in the community. We present ways that readers can advocate for people who self-injure, by adopting the person-centered framework, and learning from people with lived experience of self-injury. We hope this will encourage readers to take up the mantle and apply a strengths-based framing of self-injury in their own work and lives.

The experience of self-injury is one that is different for each and every person who self-injures. While there are some commonalities, truly understanding self-injury requires that we listen to individuals' experiences without preconceptions and without judgment. It is time to challenge the traditional deficit-based models of self-injury and to recognize the strengths, resolve, and resilience that people who self-injure possess. In doing so we avoid stigmatizing and demoralizing people who self-injure, and instead promote hope, optimism, and support seeking. Our hope is that readers find inspiration in the person-centered approach we present, and are able to take from this framework to apply a new way of thinking about self-injury that can make a significant and lasting impact for people with lived self-injury experience.

1

Self-Injury

An Overview

Before discussing the central framing guiding this book (see Chapter 3), it is first important to provide foundational knowledge about self-injury. Accordingly, this chapter addresses key areas within the field of self-injury, including how self-injury is defined, who self-injures, what might contribute to self-injury engagement, the reasons people may have for self-injury, and the risks associated with engaging in self-injury. In Chapter 2, we build on this by discussing the link between self-injury and suicide. Collectively, these two chapters provide the groundwork from which to understand and apply the person-centered, strengths-based framework woven throughout the remainder of the book.

WHAT IS SELF-INJURY?

A review of the literature points to numerous terms being used to refer to self-injury. Although having more than one term to refer to a behavior is not necessarily an issue, this becomes a concern when there is definitional inconsistency. Unfortunately, for quite some time, this is what transpired in much of the self-injury literature. We address issues of nomenclature in the next chapter as several of these terms have also been used in the context of referring to suicidal behavior.

Despite the historical confusion about what constitutes self-injury, in 2007, the International Society for the Study of Self-Injury (ISSS)—the preeminent organization in the field—put forward an official definition for nonsuicidal self-injury (NSSI; self-injury).[1] Specifically, self-injury was defined as the deliberate and self-inflicted damage to one's body tissue in the absence of suicidal intent and for reasons that are not socially or culturally sanctioned. Although "NSSI" is commonly used throughout the literature, for the purposes of simplicity and consistency, we refer to self-injury throughout the book to avoid repeated explanation of an acronym at the outset of each chapter. Thus, subsequent mention of "self-injury" in later chapters is in keeping with the above definition.

Before continuing, a few points about this definition warrant discussion. First, suicidal behaviors (which carry lethal intent) are excluded from this definition.

However, it is important to bear in mind, that while distinct, self-injury and suicide are related. Given this, we address the relation between self-injury and suicide in greater detail in the next chapter. Second, a key aspect of the above definition is the exclusion of behaviors that would be otherwise accepted in social and cultural contexts, such as tattooing and body-piercing. Finally, behaviors that can have harmful effects (e.g., substance abuse, smoking) are not included in the definition of self-injury as they do not yield *immediate* tissue damage and their adverse effects tend to occur over time.

Following the above, what behaviors are encompassed by the definition of self-injury? Although not intended to represent an exhaustive list, the most common methods of self-injury involve cutting, burning, hitting oneself (sometimes referred to as self-battery), and severe scratching/skin abrading.[2,3] Along these lines, it is important to note that there is not a prototypical method of self-injury. Rather, there is much variability with respect to how people self-injure. Further, some individuals will use just one method of self-injury, while other people will use multiple methods. In addition, how one self-injures may change over time (e.g., the initial method used may not be the method used through repeated self-injury). Because of this, it is important to avoid generalizing about how people self-injure and to instead consider people's unique experiences.

Since the inception and uptake of the aforementioned definition of self-injury, the number of empirical papers published in which the ISSS definition is used has ballooned and has steadily increased each year since.[4] It is perhaps unsurprising then that this definition mirrors the one used in the *Diagnostic and Statistical Manual for Mental* Disorders (DSM), which we discuss later in this chapter. With this growing literature in mind, we now focus the remainder of this chapter on key aspects of what we have come to learn about self-injury.

WHO SELF-INJURES?

For quite some time self-injury was primarily viewed as a symptom, and frequently an indicator, of borderline personality disorder (BPD). However, while self-injury is one of nine possible diagnostic criteria for BPD—it is neither necessary nor sufficient for one to receive such a diagnosis. Moreover, most individuals who engage in self-injury do not meet BPD criteria.[5-7] This then raises the question, who self-injures? A basic answer is that *anyone* may self-injure. But, when does self-injury tend to begin and do certain groups report more engagement in self-injury than others? We address these important questions next.

Rates and Age at Onset

The typical age at onset for self-injury is early- to mid-adolescence with another peak during early adulthood.[2,8] Although this is when self-injury most often begins it is important to bear in mind that people may start to self-injure at any age. In our own research and outreach work, we have had participants report ages at onset in early childhood and people indicating that they did not start to self-injure until well into middle and older adulthood (60+ years).[9] Indeed, individuals of *all* ages may self-injure, so it is important to avoid sweeping generalizations and misconceptions that self-injury is circumscribed to specific age groups (e.g., adolescents).

While people across the age spectrum may report self-injury, this is not to say that rates are similar across different age groups. According to a large body of research, adolescents and emerging adults consistently report the highest rates of self-injury, with up to one in five individuals in these age groups reporting self-injury at least once. More specifically, the lifetime prevalence of self-injury among adolescents typically ranges from about 13% and up to 18% in community samples.[2,10,11] Among emerging adults, rates tend to hover around 13%.[2] However, in university settings rates tend to be even higher with approximately 20% of students reporting self-injury.[2,12]

Among adults, findings from several studies have indicated that around 5.5% of adults report having self-injured on at least one occasion.[2,13] A similar but slightly lower rate (4.86%) was reported in a recent paper examining the prevalence of self-injury in a community sample of British adults.[14] Research examining self-injury among children under 12 years of age is sparser when compared to that involving other age groups. Nevertheless, some researchers have found that among children 8 to 12 years old, about 8% report having self-injured on at least one occasion.[15] Children younger than 8 may also self-injure; however, more research is needed to better understand self-injury among younger youth.

Perhaps unsurprisingly, rates among clinical samples tend to be much higher than those cited above. For instance, in some of the field's earlier published studies, self-injury rates of 40% to 61% were reported among adolescents in in-patient settings.[16,17] More recently, researchers have sought to understand rates of self-injury within particular diagnostic groups. For example, in one study about one-third of individuals diagnosed with an eating disorder reported having self-injured;[18] similar rates have been reported elsewhere, though individuals meeting criteria for bulimia nervosa (32.7%) were found to have higher rates of self-injury than individuals with anorexia nervosa (21.8%).[19] In another study examining self-injury in an inpatient sample of adolescents meeting criteria for personality disorders, the rate of self-injury was 66.4%; however, this was not circumscribed to just BPD.[20] Collectively, across the literature there are numerous reports of self-injury rates being higher when comparing a variety of samples comprising individuals from inpatient settings versus community-based settings.

In sum, adolescence and emerging adulthood represent the two age groups during which self-injury tends to begin and most often occur. However, *anyone* of *any* age may self-injure. Additionally, although self-injury rates tend to be higher among inpatient or clinical samples versus community-based samples, rates are nonetheless high in the latter. As addressed in more detail later, self-injury is transdiagnostic in nature. That is, it is not limited to a particular diagnostic group and assumptions that self-injury is a marker for borderline personality disorder— or any disorder—ought to be avoided.

Racial Diversity

Much of the empirical efforts aimed at examining the prevalence of self-injury (and studying self-injury more generally) have, to date, not sufficiently represented racially diverse populations. Of the research conducted to date, however, there is some evidence to indicate that rates of self-injury among Black, Indigenous, and People of Color (BIPOC) are higher than among white people.[21,22] However, this should not be assumed as a generality. Findings from two reviews of the literature concerning self-injury among racially diverse groups indicate that different risk (e.g., difficulties with emotion regulation, stigma) and protective factors (e.g., religion, belongingness to one's community) can influence the rate of self-injury.[21,22]

Following the above, there is a strong need in the field to work toward more diverse and equitable representation in research efforts. Doing so is an important step toward appreciating and understanding the unique and intersecting contributing factors (e.g., systemic racism; socioeconomic disadvantages) which may associate with both mental health challenges and resilience and thus influence engagement in self-injury. Thus, it is not only important to direct more efforts at understanding self-injury among racially diverse populations but also to work toward understanding the context in which self-injury occurs. Beyond working toward greater representation of diversity in terms of which populations are included in future research, efforts to enhance diversity and inclusion are not limited to *who* takes part in research but also to who conducts research. Doing so ensures historically marginalized voices are appropriately accounted for in *all* aspects of research. As this is a critical goal in the broader field and when advocating for the person-centered framework that underpins much of the book's content, we address this further in Chapter 14.

Sex, Gender, and Sexual Orientation

Previously, it was assumed that self-injury was a behavior primarily enacted by girls and women. Yet, there is now substantial evidence that the proportion of boys and men who self-injure is more or less the same.[2,5,23] The same is the case when comparing adult men and women and the proportion of individuals in these groups who report a history of self-injury.[13] This is not to say that there are no differences, however. Several studies indicate that there are differences when it comes to the behavioral features (e.g., method) of self-injury. Of note, young men tend to engage in higher rates of self-burning (including branding) and to injure on their torso/chest more often than young women; they also report self-injuring more often when under the influence of substances.[23,24] In contrast, young women tend to report more engagement in self-cutting and scratching and to report injuring their wrists and thighs.[23-25] They also tend to engage in more frequent self-injury and are more apt to talk about self-injury.[24,25]

It is important to note that many studies reporting on sex and gender differences among people who self-injure have not clearly or consistently demarcated these constructs. As a consequence, it is common to see sex-related terminology (e.g., male, female) to refer to gender and vice versa. Further, many studies have historically adopted a binary approach when reporting on sex and gender. This limits what we know with respect to sex, gender, and self-injury. Indeed, when researchers conflate sex and gender in the presentation of questions asking about participant demographic information or when binaries are used in questionnaires, individuals completing the relevant items may feel unrepresented and potentially marginalized in the research process; indeed, this can impact people's mental well-being.[26] For these reasons, it is incumbent on researchers to ensure clarity when asking about sex and gender and that the questions presented to participants are both accurate and inclusive.

Attention has increasingly been paid to understanding self-injury among lesbian, gay, bisexual, transgender, and queer (LGBTQ+) individuals as well people from gender diverse populations. Findings from a series of reviews have indicated that compared to heterosexual individuals, members of the LGBTQ+ community report higher rates of self-injury.[27-29] Relatedly, gender diverse individuals also report higher rates of self-injury when compared to their cisgender peers.[29] Much like what was mentioned in the discussion on racial diversity and self-injury, it is critical to not draw sweeping conclusions about who may be at higher risk for self-injury when considering sexual orientation and gender diverse people. Indeed, a closer look at the extant literature reveals that some groups may report higher rates of self-injury when compared to others. Specifically, both transgender and bisexual individuals report greater instances of self-injury and are considered at higher risk of self-injury.[25,29] Some research has further indicated that trans men may be at especially high risk for self-injury.[30] In line with this, transgender youth report high rates of self-injury and broader self-harm, including suicide attempts.[31]

Inasmuch as it is important to avoid generalizations about who may be at heightened risk for self-injury, it is also critical to account for the context in which self-injury occurs—that is, what may account for why members of the above groups may self-injure. While more research is needed to understand self-injury among members of the LGBTQ+ and gender diverse communities, the extant literature points to several considerations (e.g., minority stress, stigmatization because of one's sexual orientation or gender identity) that contribute to this risk.[27-29] Commensurate with attention to the context in which self-injury occurs, an array of considerations warrant attention when understanding what may lead to people engaging in self-injury. We address these in the subsequent section.

WHAT CONTRIBUTES TO SELF-INJURY?

There is significant variability and complexity with respect to what confers risk for self-injury. Indeed, there is not a single factor, nor set of factors, that consistently underlie and thus explain self-injury. Rather, multiple, and often intersecting considerations contribute to engagement in self-injury. For these reasons, no two people who engage in self-injury will be identical—even if (many) aspects of their experience are similar. Accordingly, it is essential that assumptions are avoided when it comes to what may have contributed to any one person's self-injury. Nevertheless, there are several potential risks factors for self-injury as well as risks *of* self-injury that merit discussion as they can help to better understand what may be involved in people's lived experience. Therefore, we now turn to an overview of some of the more commonly cited factors that can play a role in self-injury engagement.

Self-Injury and Mental Health Difficulties

Perhaps unsurprisingly, self-injury is associated with a wide range of mental health difficulties. Examples from several reviews and seminal texts include but are not limited to anxiety, difficulty with coping and managing emotion, self-criticism, impulsivity, and negative body image.[5,32–36] Similarly, self-injury can also occur in the context of mental disorders. But, as previously mentioned, self-injury is not limited to specific forms of mental disorders, such as BPD, as was previously thought. Indeed, self-injury has been found to co-occur with eating disorders, major depression, post-traumatic stress disorder, and substance abuse, among other forms of mental illness.[5,32–39] Thus, self-injury is transdiagnostic in nature. Importantly, although it is the case that self-injury is associated with an array of mental disorders, just because someone self-injures does not mean that a mental disorder is present. Many individuals will self-injure but not meet criteria for a mental disorder.[5,32–35]

Outside of its association with both mental health difficulties and mental disorders, self-injury has also been found to share a relation with numerous adversities and difficult life events. For example, self-injury has been shown to correlate with having attachment difficulties, parental criticism, and parent loss.[5,32–35] For quite some time it was also presumed that self-injury was the manifestation of childhood trauma—in particular, childhood sexual abuse.[40–44] Research, however, has indicated otherwise.[34,45] Certainly, self-injury associates with trauma, including childhood sexual abuse; in other words, people who have experienced such trauma are at elevated risk for self-injury. However, trauma in the form of childhood sexual abuse is not a unique predictor of self-injury.[34,45] Rather, researchers have demonstrated that this link is better accounted for by depression, post-traumatic symptoms, and other interpersonal factors.[39,45] Engagement in self-injury also associates with other forms of trauma (e.g., emotional and physical abuse, bullying), yet the presence of self-injury should not signal that one has a history of trauma.[5,32–35] Not all individuals who self-injure necessarily have these experiences.[5,32–35]

Self-Injury as a Standalone Diagnosis

There have been many cases made to have self-injury included as a formal diagnosis, much like major depression or post-traumatic stress disorder.[46-50] Although initial efforts did not result in the inclusion of self-injury within the diagnostic nomenclature this changed in 2013, with the publication of the Fifth Edition of the *Diagnostic and Statistical Manual of Mental Disorders* (DSM-5). Although not technically a mental disorder, Non-Suicidal Self-Injury Disorder was included in Section 3 of the DSM-5 as a condition warranting further research.[51] Box 1.1 outlines the proposed criteria for NSSI Disorder.

Box 1.1

PROPOSED DIAGNOSTIC CRITERIA FOR NONSUICIDAL SELF-INJURY DISORDER.

A. In last year, the individual has, on ≥ 5 days, engaged in intentional self-inflicted damage to the surface of body of a sort likely to induce bleeding, bruising, or pain (e.g., cutting, burning, stabbing, hitting, excessive rubbing), with the expectation that the injury will lead to minor-moderate physical harm (i.e., no suicidal intent).

B. The individual engages in the self-injurious behavior with one or more of the following expectations:
1. To obtain relief from negative feeling/cognitive state.
2. To resolve an interpersonal difficulty.
3. To induce a positive feeling state.

C. The intentional self-injury associated with ≥1 of:
1. Interpersonal difficulties or negative feelings or thoughts occurring immediately prior to the act.
2. Prior to engaging in the act, a period of preoccupation with the intended behavior that is difficult to control.
3. Thinking about self-injury that occurs frequently, even when it is not acted upon.

D. Not socially sanctioned or limited to scab-picking, nail biting.

E. Behavior or its consequences cause significant distress or interference in key areas of functioning.

F. Not limited to psychotic episodes, delirium, substances. In neurodevelopmental dx, behavior not repetitive stereotypy. Not better explained by other mental/medical condition.

Pursuant to this, much research has examined the utility, reliability, and validity of the proposed DSM-5 criteria for NSSI Disorder.[46,49,50,52-54] Evidence from these efforts have demonstrated that the proposed NSSI Disorder can be meaningfully differentiated from other mental disorders such as BPD.[49,53,55,56] and that many of the criteria carry research and clinical usefulness.[46] Collectively, there appears to be a growing likelihood that NSSI Disorder will be formally incorporated in a future revision to the DSM.[52,54,55,57]

Despite the many studies investigating NSSI Disorder, it is critical to consider how individuals with lived experience view the prospect of self-injury being diagnosed as a mental disorder. Some of our research has shown that people with lived experience see both advantages and disadvantages about this.[58] Among the potential advantages, people who self-injure highlight the possibility that NSSI Disorder being included in the DSM could result in greater understanding of self-injury (e.g., through more research funding). They also indicate that this may work to legitimize people's experience and enhance both help-seeking and treatment. Regarding the disadvantages, however, some individuals with lived experience have expressed caution that inclusion of self-injury as a diagnostic category may foment stigma and undermine the many factors underlying self-injury—including those discussed in this chapter. Thus, if (and seemingly when) self-injury is adopted as a formal mental disorder, it will be vital that researchers and clinicians work to address these concerns.

REASONS FOR SELF-INJURY

As we unpack further in Chapter 4, self-injury is unfortunately and commonly stigmatized.[59] One of the many consequences of this are particular myths and misconceptions regarding why people self-injure. Perhaps the most common of these is that self-injury is inaccurately viewed as attention-seeking and manipulative in nature.[60,61] These views are in sharp contrast to a robust literature—including comprehensive review papers—that points to myriad reasons for self-injury.[62,63] Furthermore, rendering self-injury attention-seeking and manipulative is reductionistic and unhelpful, as these views place fault and blame on the individual (e.g., for doing something wrong or that they should not) and fail to capture the context in which self-injury occurs.

A review of the literature highlights that there are numerous reasons for self-injury (see Table 1.1). Most often these have been conceptualized as falling into two overarching categories, namely intrapersonal reasons and social (or interpersonal) reasons for the behavior. Of these, there is significant evidence that intrapersonal reasons are more commonly reported. Along these lines, by and large, the most frequently cited reason that people give for self-injury is that it is used to obtain temporary relief from *unwanted* and often intense and very painful emotional experiences.[63] In other words, self-injury is used as a coping strategy. Indeed, many people report that in response to strong emotions (e.g., anxiety,

Table 1.1. COMMON INTRAPERSONAL AND SOCIAL REASONS FOR SELF-INJURY
(THIS IS NOT INTENDED TO BE AN EXHAUSTIVE LIST).

Examples of Intrapersonal Reasons	Examples of Social Reasons
To cope with and obtain relief from intense emotional experiences (e.g., distress, anxiety)	To communicate that one is in pain or struggling to cope
To punish oneself and express self-criticism or self-loathing	To communicate a need for support
To stop feeling dissociated, depersonalized, or emotionally numb; to feel something when feeling numb or dissociated; to "feel real"	To demonstrate toughness to others
To avoid acting on suicidal thoughts or urges	

distress, sadness) they turn to self-injury, which yields ephemeral relief from these states.

Supporting the view of self-injury as a coping strategy is a substantial body of research.[62,63] This entails a corpus of self-report studies[64-66] as well as lab-based studies in which findings indicate that both people who have and who have not self-injured experience less aversive emotion following exposure to a pain-inducing task.[67-69] In concert with this, there is empirical support that pain can be effective in alleviating difficult emotions. This is especially the case for individuals who report more self-criticism, which is both common and typically higher among people who self-injure.[70,71] It is therefore understandable that individuals who engage in self-injury will turn to self-injury during instances of emotional pain. Indeed, self-injury works to cope with these experiences, as it reduces intense and difficult emotions. Before discussing other reasons for self-injury, while emotional pain is typically implicated in the context of self-injury engagement, it should not be assumed that this is the only emotional experience preceding self-injury. A range of emotions may also occur prior to self-injury (e.g., frustration, anger, sadness, anxiety).[62,63]

Perhaps the second most common reason reported for self-injury is to punish oneself or to express self-loathing.[62,63] As alluded to earlier, many individuals with lived experience of self-injury report high levels of self-criticism; correspondingly, it is not uncommon for people to also report hating themselves.[72] In these cases, self-injury may be used to either demonstrate or express self-criticism or self-loathing. At the same time, self-injury may be similarly used to cope with these intense and potentially overwhelming emotional experiences. Hence, self-injury may serve more than one purpose at a given time.

Beyond these intrapersonal reasons for self-injury, others warrant some attention. Among these is that for some people, self-injury is used to alleviate feelings of dissociation, depersonalization, or emotional numbness. It may also be used to generate a feeling during these psychological states (e.g., to feel real or alive versus feeling numb). Additionally, self-injury may serve as a means to mitigate suicidal thoughts and to avoid acting on them.[62]

Finally, as mentioned earlier, self-injury may be engaged in for interpersonal reasons. Although typically less frequently reported, this can involve self-injuring to communicate pain or a need for help, to establish boundaries between the self and others, and to signal toughness to others.[62,64,65] Because self-injury can have interpersonal reasons, this may also help to explain—though not excuse—some of the myths regarding self-injury, notably those mentioned earlier such as self-injury being misconstrued as a form of attention-seeking or manipulation. For example, an attempt to communicate that one is in emotional pain through an act of self-injury may be dismissed as attention-seeking. However, for some people, it may be immensely difficult to articulate how much pain they are experiencing; they may not know how to do this. Hence, self-injury may be used to express the gravity of their pain, only for this to be viewed in stigmatizing or otherwise un-helpful ways.

At this point, it should be clear that people self-injure for many different reasons. Along these lines, there are several considerations to keep in mind when understanding why people self-injure; these are summarized in Box 1.2. First, while we have focused on the more frequently cited reasons in the literature, the reasons discussed thus far should not be viewed as an exhaustive list. Indeed, people may have other reasons for self-injury. Second, people may self-injure for more than one reason. On the one hand, this may mean that the reason for self-injury may differ across contexts; it may be that self-injury serves more than one purpose at a given time. For example, people may self-injure in response to in-tense self-criticism to both express how they feel but also obtain relief from the pain that comes with this view of self. Third, the initial reason(s) for self-injury may differ from those involved in its repetition. For instance, someone might in-itially self-injure to cope with emotional pain but later use the behavior to avoid acting on suicidal urges. Thus, people's reasons may change, and these changes may occur at different points (i.e., not limited to the initial onset and then repeti-tion of self-injury).

Box 1.2

SUMMARY OF KEY CONSIDERATIONS REGARDING REASONS FOR SELF-INJURY.

Reasons for Self-injury: Key Considerations

Although people most often report using self-injury to cope with painful
 emotions, this should not be assumed. There are many reasons for self-injury.
People often self-injure for more than one reason.
The initial reason for self-injury may differ from the reason(s) self-injury
 continues.
Reasons for self-injury may vary across contexts and time.
People may have difficulty explaining why they self-injure (e.g., due to stigma,
 not knowing how to express underlying difficulties).

It is also important to bear in mind that sometimes individuals may have difficulty expressing *why* they self-injure. This is understandable. It can be hard to share experiences that are painful or that are stigmatized, and it can be difficult for people without lived experience to fully understand why someone might intentionally hurt themselves. One final note regarding reasons for self-injury pertains to how people describe why they self-injure. Much of what we summarize in this section of the chapter comes from research using questionnaires or interviews that ask direct questions about why someone might self-injure. However, the language used in these approaches may not perfectly align with how someone might describe their experience. Therefore, when trying to understand someone's reasons for self-injury, situating them as an expert in their own experience and actively listening to their description of what self-injury does for them is essential.

CONSEQUENCES OF SELF-INJURY

Beyond what may contribute to initial and continued self-injury, there is also a range of consequences that stem from self-injury itself. Certainly, by virtue of engaging in self-injury, individuals are at risk for a range of injury types which will vary based on the self-injury method and medical severity. Relatedly, self-injury may result in residual scarring. A growing body of research indicates that scarring from self-injury is highly salient among many people with lived experience. For example, it may play a role in the context of recovery as well as in the stigmatization of self-injury.[73-76] In line with scarring being involved in the context of stigma, self-injury, in general, can evoke significant stigma.[59] In this way, individuals who self-injure may experience stigma from others as well as internalized stigma. For these reasons, we address stigma and recovery in a more fulsome manner in Chapters 4 and 11, respectively. Outside of this, individuals who engage in self-injury are also at greater risk for suicide. Given the centrality of this risk and the import of understanding how self-injury and suicide are interrelated, we dedicate the next chapter to this topic.

SUMMARY

Notwithstanding the documented myths and misunderstandings concerning self-injury, the significant strides in research over the past decade or so have vastly increased our understanding of self-injury. These collective research efforts have established that self-injury is a common, serious, but highly complex behavior. Numerous factors can contribute to self-injury and each person's experience will be, to varying degrees, unique. Likewise, people may have different reasons for self-injury (with some people having more than one reason or reasons that change over time). Given this, and congruent with recent shifts in the field, a person-centered approach—that emphasizes people's lived experience—is needed when understanding self-injury and in the context of supporting people who self-injure.[77-80] In our view, doing so is paramount to ensuring people with lived experience are supported and understood. Hence, we have structured this book to facilitate and deepen how self-injury is understood while also providing practical information that can promote greater well-being and better outcomes for people with lived experience.

Self-Injury and Suicidal Thoughts and Behaviors

AN ISSUE OF TERMINOLOGY

Historically, exploration of self-inflicted harm has been hampered by definitional inconsistency and ambiguity. In fact, self-injury holds the unfortunate position of having countless terms used to describe a behavior. Among the terms used throughout the literature are: "self-mutilation," "self-inflicted violence," "self-abuse," "deliberate self-harm," "self-harm" (with the "deliberate" qualifier seen as implicit), "nonsuicidal self-injury," "self-injury," and "parasuicide." In some cases, self-injury has simply been referred to as cutting, fostering the misunderstanding that cutting is the only form of self-injury. Terms such as "self-mutilation" and "parasuicide" quickly fell out of favor as they were considered pejorative, and seen as unhelpful by people with lived experience of these behaviors.

Today, the terms "self-harm" and "non-suicidal self-injury" (NSSI or simply "self-injury") are more commonly used. Yet there is still confusion regarding which behaviors constitute self-harm. For some, self-harm means any nonfatal, self-inflicted behavior irrespective of intent (including suicide attempts[1]); others include only behaviors enacted without conscious suicidal intent.[2] As seen in Figure 2.1, self-harm might best be conceptualized as a broad umbrella term that encompasses self-injury, poisoning, suicide attempts, and culturally or socially appropriate forms of harm (e.g., religious or cultural practices). To aid in the differentiation of these behaviors, the International Society for the Study of Self-Injury[2] explicitly defined self-injury as the deliberate, self-inflicted damage to body tissue *without suicidal intent*, and for purposes not socially or culturally sanctioned. While intent can be difficult to determine, and fluctuates over time,[3] failure to make this distinction can result in inaccurate risk assessment, inappropriate treatment, and unnecessary hospitalization.[4] For these reasons, throughout this book, we focus our attention specifically on self-injury.

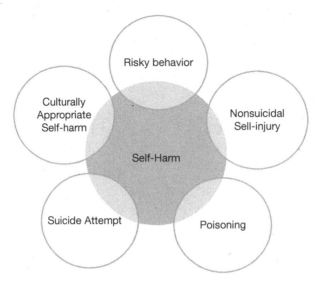

Figure 2.1. Conceptualization of self-harm.

SIMILARITIES AND DIFFERENCES BETWEEN SELF-INJURY AND SUICIDAL BEHAVIORS

On the surface, self-injury and suicidal behaviors can appear quite similar. Both are deliberate acts of damage against the self. Both have been associated with severe psychological distress and mental illness, including major depression, anxiety disorders, and substance use disorders.[5] Both self-injury and suicide attempts are more common among females (although death by suicide is more common among males). Although we do not have accurate epidemiological data, some studies report that among people who report a suicide attempt, 68% also report a history of self-injury.[6] Similarly, some studies report that among people who engage in self-injury, 33% report a prior suicide attempt,[7] suggesting some overlap across the behaviors.

At the same time, there are many differences that support the idea that self-injury and suicidal behaviors are distinct. The primary distinction is the intention underlying the behavior; self-injury is usually engaged as a means of coping with distressing or upsetting emotional states while suicidal behaviors are engaged as a means of ending life.[5] In other words, one is used to cope with adversities in life and the other is engaged with the intention of ending life. Not surprisingly then, self-injury is engaged more often than suicidal behaviors, has an earlier age of onset, and usually involves less lethal means (e.g., skin cutting vs. hanging[5]).

HOW ARE SELF-INJURY AND SUICIDAL BEHAVIOR RELATED?

In line with the definitional ambiguity, there has been ongoing debate in the literature as to whether self-injury and suicidal acts are truly separate behaviors, or whether they exist on a continuum of self-harming behavior, with self-injury at the less severe end of the spectrum and suicide attempts at the most severe. Proponents of a continuum approach argue that self-injury typically precedes suicidal thoughts and behaviors, but that when the underlying distress is not resolved, more lethal means of self-harm are used to permanently end the distress.[8] In this way, self-injury is seen as a gateway to suicidal thoughts and behaviors, similar to how marijuana use is perceived to be a gateway to use of more harmful illicit drugs. Supporters of the notion that the behaviors are separate point to the fact that suicidal thoughts and behaviors can fluctuate, and that people can, and do, engage in both suicidal and nonsuicidal behaviors across the lifespan.[5] Further, the two behaviors differ in a number of features, including descriptive features (e.g., means of injury), demographic characteristics (e.g., gender), and psychosocial variables (suicidal behavior is accompanied by a sense of hopelessness rather than one of trying to cope with life).[5]

Another point of view is that there is a common third variable (or set of variables) that underlies both self-injury and suicidal behavior.[5] Both self-injury and suicidal behavior are associated with psychological distress and psychological disorders, which may themselves increase risk for both behaviors. However, research comparing individuals who report self-injury, individuals who report a suicide attempt, and individuals who report both, shows that these groups can be differentiated on levels of distress and mental illness. If these factors were the cause of both self-injury and suicidal behavior, the psychological profiles would be similar.

Bringing all these conceptualizations together, Hamza and colleagues[5] proposed an integrated model. In particular, they clearly differentiate self-injury and suicidal behavior, but suggest a direct link between self-injury and suicidal behavior (consistent with the Gateway theory). They also propose that this relation may be impacted by additional variables common to both behaviors (consistent with the third variable model). Finally, they outline a role for acquired capability for suicide, consistent with Joiner's interpersonal theory of suicide[9] (discussed in detail below). In doing so, Hamza and her colleagues propose that we do not need to adhere to any one conceptualization of the association between self-injury and suicidal behavior, but that all accounts warrant consideration.

HOW DO WE EXPLAIN THE RELATION BETWEEN SELF-INJURY AND SUICIDAL THOUGHTS AND BEHAVIORS?

Perhaps the most widely used theory linking self-injury and suicidal behavior is Joiner's interpersonal theory of suicide.[9] Joiner proposed that in order to die by suicide an individual must have both a desire to suicide and the ability to take their own life. Contributing to the desire to die by suicide are an unmet need to belong, termed "thwarted belongingness", and perceiving oneself to be a burden on others, termed "perceived burdensomeness." Both thwarted belonging and perceived burdensomeness are considered to be multifaceted constructs that encompass a number of known risk factors for suicide (e.g., loneliness, child abuse,

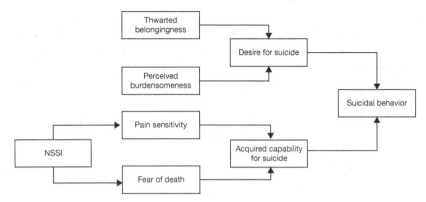

Figure 2.2. Joiner's interpersonal model of suicide.

loss of loved ones, family conflict, unemployment, homelessness, self-hate, low self-esteem; see Figure 2.2).

The ability to take one's life is referred to as acquired capability for suicide. Joiner proposes that in order to feel one is capable of taking their own life they need to lose the fear of death, and have a capacity to endure pain that may arise from the means of suicide.[10] As humans, we are evolutionary programed to strive for life and avoid life-threatening situations. When exploring reasons for living, many cite a fear of death as a reason they do not attempt suicide. As such, the ability to take one's life requires that enough of this fear has dissipated that it no longer presents a barrier to suicide. In addition, methods of suicide often involve physical pain. To have the capability to die by suicide an individual needs to be able to withstand this self-inflicted pain. Pain tolerance is something that varies widely from individual to individual, yet there is reliable evidence that individuals who have engaged in self-injury have a higher tolerance for pain than individuals with no history of self-injury or suicidal behavior.[11] Of course, an individual may have a different tolerance for different types of pain, and this likely informs the means of suicide an individual will choose.

Joiner uses the concepts of habituation and opponent processes to explain how someone may develop acquired capability for suicide over time.[9] With repeated exposure to fearful or painful experiences one's level of fear and pain tend to dissipate; this is known as habituation. Opponent process theory suggests that emotional responses often comprise two competing (or opponent) processes. For example, a fear of suicide may also be accompanied by a sense of anticipated relief or escape. With repeated exposure the primary process (fear) tends to reduce while the strength of the opponent process (escape) is amplified. To demonstrate how habituation and opponent processes work together, Van Orden and colleagues use the example of an individual who goes bungee jumping. Their initial reaction is likely to be one of fear (primary process). However, with repeated exposure this fear will reduce and the opponent process of exhilaration will increase.[10]

Of note, Joiner mentions self-injury as one factor that, through repeated acts, can increase the capability for suicide. Specifically, he argues that the initial response (primary process) to self-injury may be fear and an expectation of pain. However, self-injury also produces emotional relief (the opponent process). Over time, self-injury becomes less fearful, and the association with emotional relief becomes stronger. Repeated self-injury may also increase pain tolerance, as an individual becomes more comfortable with deliberately hurting themselves.[9]

Supporting this theory, people who repeatedly self-injure feel calmer and more relieved following self-injury than people who self-injure less frequently, suggesting the opponent process of relief becomes more reinforcing with greater repetition of the behavior.[12] In experimental tasks, people who self-injure generally endure painful stimuli for longer than people who do not self-injure,[13] and the relation between self-injury and suicide attempts is stronger for people with high levels of pain persistence.[14] After conducting a meta-analysis of prior studies, Koenig and colleagues[11] noted that individuals who engage in self-injury exhibit a greater pain threshold, greater pain tolerance, and lower pain intensity compared to individuals who do not self-injure.

Among college students, self-injury prospectively predicts acquired capability for suicide.[15] In a direct test of the model among sexual minority youth, Muehlenkamp and colleagues[16] found that self-injury was related to suicidal thoughts and behaviors, working though acquired capability. Extending the original model, Chu and colleagues[17] noted that self-injury was also associated with thwarted belongingness and perceived burdensomeness among young adults. Further, self-injury prospectively predicted suicide ideation, through perceived burdensomeness. Similar patterns have been observed among military service members and veterans.[18] The link between self-injury and acquired capability has become so accepted that many researchers use measures of self-injury as a proxy for acquired capability for suicide.[19,20]

DOES SELF-INJURY INCREASE RISK OF LATER SUICIDAL THOUGHTS AND BEHAVIORS?

Although a link between self-injury and suicidal thoughts and behaviors is commonly accepted, there are very few longitudinal studies that allow us to determine whether self-injury is a unique risk factor for later suicide. In one study with adolescents, a history of self-injury conferred a threefold risk in concurrent or later suicidal thoughts or behaviors, with youth who engaged in 20 or more acts of self-injury most at risk.[8] Among college students, a prior history of self-injury is associated with a 5.5 times greater risk of a subsequent suicide attempt.[21] This risk is increased to 330 times the risk for students who meet proposed DSM-5 criteria for Non-Suicidal Self-Injury Disorder.[22] Thoughts of self-injury, in the absence of the behavior itself, are associated with later suicide ideation and making a plan for suicide. Further, self-injury differentiates students who report suicide ideation and act on these thoughts from those who do not attempt suicide.[22] Consistent with Whitlock's work with adolescents, young adults who engage in more than 20 acts of self-injury are at increased risk of suicide attempt. In clinical samples, frequency of self-injury appears to predict subsequent suicide attempts, with more frequent self-injury increasing risk of later suicide attempt.[23]

In a meta-analysis of risk factors for suicide, Franklin and colleagues[24] observed self-injury to be the most reliable predictor of a suicide attempt; individuals reporting a history of self-injury were four times more likely to report an attempt than individuals who had no self-injury history. However, the authors also noted that predictive effects were quite weak and caution against using any one predictor as an indicator of suicide risk. When specifically analyzing studies reporting on the relation between self-injurious thoughts and behaviors, and future suicide ideation, attempts, and death, Ribeiro and colleagues[25] again observed that self-injury was the most reliable predictor of later suicide attempts. However overall prediction was weak, with individuals reporting a history of self-injury only twice as likely as those without a history to later record a suicide attempt.

In sum, it seems that people who self-injure are more likely to report suicidal thoughts and behaviors than individuals with no history of self-injury, whether this be in the past, concurrent with self-injury, or in the future. However, there is no accurate data on just how many people who self-injure will engage in future suicidal thoughts and behaviors. The statistical modeling that has been conducted suggests there is a reliable association between self-injury and future suicide risk, however this effect is small, and self-injury should not be used as the sole indicator of suicide risk.

A PERSON-CENTERED APPROACH

It may be apparent from reading this chapter that the link between self-injury and suicidal thoughts and behaviors is complex. Issues with terminology, consideration of the overlap between self-injury and suicidal behavior, as well as the important distinctions, and a lack of solid evidence regarding the prospective relation between self-injury and later suicidal behavior all hinder understanding of this relationship. However, despite these concerns, the research consistently points to elevated rates of suicidal thoughts and behavior among people with a history of self-injury. For this reason, consideration of suicide risk is important when supporting someone who self-injures.

To ensure a complete understanding of an individual's experience it is important to focus on each instance of self-inflicted harm, rather than assume the motives and functions of all acts of harm are the same. As noted earlier, suicidal thoughts can fluctuate over time, and while one act of self-injury may be nonsuicidal in nature, a later act may be underpinned by thoughts of suicide. Likewise, someone who has attempted suicide may subsequently engage in nonsuicidal self-injury. Rather than making assumptions, it is critical to adopt a person-centered approach to ask the individual what is going on for them, at that time. Individuals can adopt a *respectful curiosity* to empathically enquire about their experience.[26] Here, a genuine interest in understanding one's lived experience with self-injury is communicated. This approach is particularly effective as it conveys a genuine commitment to wanting to understand what self-injury, or suicidal thoughts and behaviors, mean for the individual.

Given fluctuations in suicidal thoughts and behaviors, it is important to ask about suicide, and if necessary conduct a suicide risk assessment. Ongoing monitoring of suicidal thoughts and behaviors—without over monitoring—is warranted. Many people become anxious talking about suicide, afraid that talking about it will increase risk for vulnerable people. However, this is not true. Instead, talking about suicide opens the doors to better communication and fosters support seeking for someone who is currently struggling.[27] One could start by simply asking, "Do you ever have thoughts of suicide when you self-injure? What about at other times?" The response to this question is likely to determine the level of care or intervention required. Avoid minimizing the person's feeling (e.g., "You have everything to live for"), or promoting stigma (e.g., "Suicide is selfish," "People who die by suicide are weak and just can't handle life"). The important thing is that you take the time to listen to what is going on for this person, at this time.

In talking about suicide, or suicidal thoughts, the language we use is important.[28] Like self-injury, suicide carries significant stigma, and it is important to ensure the language used does not further promote or worsen stigma. Terms such as "committed suicide" associate suicide with criminal acts or being involuntarily committed to a mental institution, and risk stigmatizing both the person who dies by suicide and those bereaved by the death. Instead, use terms such as "died by suicide" or talk about someone who "took their own life." Likewise, when considering suicide attempts avoid terms such as "failed suicide attempt" or "unsuccessful suicide," which have an emphasis on failure (see Table 2.1). For

Table 2.1. PRACTICAL TIPS REGARDING LANGUAGE AND ASKING ABOUT SUICIDAL THOUGHTS AND BEHAVIORS.

Language to avoid	Instead use
• Commit suicide	• Died by suicide
• Successful suicide	• Took their own life
• Failed suicide	• Attempted to end their life
• Unsuccessful suicide	• Nonfatal attempt

Questions to ask about suicidal thoughts and behaviors
- Do you ever have thoughts of suicide when you self-injure? What about at other times?
- How much do you feel like acting on these thoughts right now?
- Why do you think you feel this way?
- I know that talking about suicidal thoughts or feelings can be hard. Know that I am here when you are ready to talk.
- Have you thought about how you would end your life? (The point here is not to focus on the method, but to determine if the individual has a suicide plan, which indicates increased risk)
- Have you thought about talking to a professional to help with these feelings? I can come with you if you like.
- What can I do to help?

the individual who survives an attempt this could be construed as one more thing they were not able to achieve, and could exacerbate a sense of hopelessness—a key factor in risk for suicide. Instead, talk about someone who has "attempted to take their life."

DEVELOPING A SAFETY PLAN

The gold-standard approach to preventing suicide among people experiencing suicide ideation is to develop a safety plan.[29] A safety plan may also be a useful tool to help people engaging in self-injury—whether this is accompanied by suicidal thoughts or not. When people feel particularly distressed it can be difficult to think about alternate coping strategies. The distress or emotional pain can feel overwhelming, and people can develop "tunnel vision," seeing self-injury or suicide as the only solution. Developing a safety, or support, plan provides individuals with strategies to help them see other options they could use instead of self-injury or suicide (see Table 2.2).

Taking a person-centered approach, a safety plan is individually tailored for the person, and does not make assumptions about their experiences. Safety plans can be completed alone, or with the help of a friend, or mental health professional. When developing a safety plan it is important that the individual finds a time

Table 2.2. SAMPLE SAFETY PLAN TO BE INDIVIDUALLY TAILORED (BY FILLING IN THE EXTRA SPACE).

Safety Plan Components

Warning signs

Keeping safe

Reasons for living (or not engaging in self-injury)

Alternative coping strategies

Family and friends I can turn to

Name:	Phone number:
Name:	Phone number:
Name:	Phone number:

Professional supports

Name:	Phone number:
Name:	Phone number:
Name:	Phone number:

when they are calm, and are in a safe place, that allows them to clearly think about their self-injury and alternative strategies that could be used. The first step of safety planning involves recognizing an individual's warning signs. These are potential triggers that increase risk of self-injury or suicidal behavior. These might be a fight with a loved one, poor performance at school or work, or just a build-up of many little stressors over time. The second step is to ensure the individual's environment is safe. In the case of suicide safety planning this might mean restricting access to means to suicide. With self-injury this is a little more difficult, as almost anything can be used to self-injure. However, some people might find that limiting access to their preferred means of self-injury may reduce their engagement in the behavior. Next, the person outlines reasons they do not want to self-injure. These might be short-term or long-term reasons, but will serve as a reminder when urges are strong that the individual has identified reasons that they do not want to self-injure. Many people report ambivalence about wanting to completely stop self-injury, recognizing that it is an effective, although not ideal, way to alleviate distress.[30,31] A reason not to engage in self-injury might be as simple as "I do not want to self-injure *at this point in my life*," which does not take self-injury off the table indefinitely, but may give someone the motivation they need to resist an urge to self-injure in that moment. The impact self-injury has on family and friends is also commonly reported as a reason not to engage in the behavior.

An important step of safety planning is to identify alternate coping strategies. As noted above, when feeling distressed it can be really difficult to think of other strategies that have worked in the past and self-injury (or suicide) can seem like the only viable option for managing, avoiding, or escaping distress. Writing down a list of alternatives that have previously worked means the person does not need to think of them while distressed—they are already written down, and can serve as reminders of what else has worked in the past. Touching base with family and friends, even if it is just to vent, can be important to re-establish that sense of belonging and gain social support. Finally, the individual should write down a list of professional resources and supports that they can call on if things get really bad. Again, having these at hand means not needing to look them up during a period of heightened distress.

CONCLUSION

Although not engaged with conscious suicidal intent, self-injury and suicidal thoughts and behaviors often do co-occur. Moreover, self-injury is the most reliable predictor of later suicidal thoughts and behaviors. Adopting a person-centered approach means acknowledging that an individual may engage in a range of self-harming behaviors, for different reasons at different times. Compassionately asking about suicidal thoughts provides a space for open communication, without judgment, and may foster understanding of an individual's experience. Developing a safety plan may be one strategy an individual could use, both to limit use of self-injury or to avoid acting on suicidal urges.

A Person-Centered, Strengths-Based Framing of Self-Injury

THEORETICAL MODELS OF SELF-INJURY

Experiential Avoidance Model

One of the first efforts to explain the initiation and maintenance of self-injury, the experiential avoidance model[1] posits that self-injury is maintained by a cycle of negative reinforcement, through the avoidance of unwanted emotional experiences. Central to this model is the idea that individuals have varying degrees to which they can sit with their emotions, or wish to avoid them. Individuals who self-injure are thought to be more likely to want to avoid intense or unwanted emotions. As such, unwanted emotional experiences are likely to trigger this desire to avoid them, and self-injury is used as a means of doing this. Further, the relation between the unwanted emotion and avoidance can be amplified or attenuated by an individual's levels of distress tolerance, emotional intensity, and emotion regulation.

Nock's Integrated Model of Self-Injury

Matthew Nock's[2] integrated theoretical model of the development and maintenance of self-injury considers risk factors for self-injury as well as factors that maintain the behavior. Both distal (e.g., genetic predisposition) and proximal (e.g., stressful events) are considered, as are intra- and interpersonal vulnerability factors, such as poor communication skills and poor distress tolerance. Nock asserts that self-injury can be reinforced either by regulation of one's emotion or by regulation of a social situation. Unique to Nock's model is the presentation of a number of self-injury-specific vulnerability factors. These are hypotheses regarding why someone may engage in self-injury rather than an alternative behavior and include: modeling the behavior from others, self-punishment, communicating distress, the ease with which self-injury can be engaged and the effectiveness of the behavior, reduced pain sensitivity, and identifying as someone who self-injures.

Emotional Cascade Model

The emotional cascade model[3] was developed as a means of explaining the occurrence of dysregulated behaviors, like self-injury, in the context of borderline personality disorder. Central to this model is the notion that intensely ruminating on negative emotion can amplify the emotional experience. This can develop into an "emotional cascade" whereby continued rumination leads to increasingly intense emotion. Ultimately, the emotion reaches an intensity that cannot be downregulated through coping strategies such as listening to music or going for a walk, but requires a strategy that matches the intensity of the emotion and allows the cycle to be interrupted. Self-injury achieves this by distracting from the cycle of rumination and emotion, as the individual focuses on the injury, the sight or blood, wound care, or other aspects of self-injury.

Cognitive-Emotional Model

The cognitive-emotion model[4] builds on prior emotion-focused theories of self-injury to incorporate elements of social cognitive theory.[5] Specifically, the model allows for anticipated consequences of the behavior to feature in the decision to self-injure. That is, outcome expectancies, or what a person believes will happen if they self-injure, operate to guide behavior, with anticipated positive consequences increasing likelihood of self-injury and anticipated negative consequences decreasing likelihood of the behavior.[6] These cognitions are coupled with an individual's beliefs about their ability to deliberately hurt themselves, and their beliefs in their ability to resist acting on urges to self-injure. An individual brings these beliefs to any given situation, and when in an emotionally volatile situation their tendency to ruminate or reappraise the situation will underpin the intensity of the emotional response. Here, self-injury may be used to avoid the situation itself, or to avoid the emotional experience. The existence or effectiveness of alternative emotion regulation strategies then determines whether self-injury may be used to down (or up) regulate the emotional response.

Benefits and Barriers Model

The benefits and barriers model[7] is unique in recognizing the self-injury offers several advantages to individuals who engage in the behavior. These include the

relief when pain is ceased, emotion regulation and/or self-punishment, peer affiliation for some, and communication of distress or strength. Yet, a number of
barriers are proposed to act to prevent individuals from capitalizing on these
benefits. These include a lack of awareness of self-injury, aversion to pain, aversion to self-injury stimuli (e.g., the sight of blood), a positive view of the self, and
anticipated negative reactions from others.

LIMITS OF EXISTING MODELS

All of these models have allowed us to make significant advancements in our
understanding of factors that are related to the initiation and maintenance of
self-injury. All have led to extensive research efforts, which have supported the
theoretical underpinning of each model, and identified targets for intervention
(e.g., increasing distress tolerance, emotion regulation). However, all of these
models, with perhaps the exception of the benefits and barriers model, are
deficit-based models. That is, they all emphasize areas in which an individual
who self-injures is lacking. Individuals who self-injure are proposed to have
limited or *infective* emotion regulation strategies, are *unable* to tolerate distress, tend to *avoid* emotion, and so forth. This focus on deficits can be demoralizing for individuals who self-injure, and reinforce deficit-based messages
they have likely already been exposed to through media and discussions with
others. While efforts to increase emotional awareness and learn alternative
coping strategies may be warranted and ultimately helpful for many people,
these models fail to explicitly recognize the many strengths that individuals
who self-injure possess.

There are a number of potential unintended consequences of adopting medical,
or deficits-based, models to understand self-injury. These include the potential to
increase or perpetuate stigma through the use of language that may be hurtful or
promulgate stereotypes[8-10] and the inappropriate conceptualization of self-injury
recovery[11-12]—both of which we discuss later in this book. In light of this we advocate for inclusion of individuals with lived experience in research and clinical
efforts,[13] and the adoption of a person-centered approach when understanding
someone's lived experience of self-injury.[14]

STRENGTHS-BASED APPROACHES

Borrowing from the field of positive psychology, strengths-based approaches
focus on identifying an individual's strengths and building resilience, rather than
focusing on weaknesses or areas of deficit. In this way, an individual learns to build
confidence and self-esteem, which can help in all aspects of their lives. A recent
meta-analysis provides support for strengths-based interventions in decreasing
symptoms of depression and increasing life satisfaction.[15]

Padesky and Mooney[16] suggest a four-step process to strengths-based cognitive therapy. These include:

1. Identifying strengths
2. Constructing a personal model of resilience
3. Applying this personalized model to difficulties in life
4. Practicing resilience

A pilot trial of this approach evidenced significant improvements in distress, self-esteem, optimism, and quality of life among college students.[17] Strengths can be identified in a number of different ways, but are most often recorded with the Values in Action Inventory of Strengths[18] (see Chapter 12). This inventory outlines core values a person possesses with matching character strengths, which provides numerous opportunities for individuals to identify strengths in different aspects of their lives.

To the best of our knowledge, a strengths-based approach has not been applied directly to understanding self-injury. In an early feasibility study, we explored the views of school staff regarding a solution-focused program designed to reduce self-injury. Solutions-focused approaches are also housed in the field of positive psychology, and are related to strengths-based approaches in that they foster development of a range of coping skills and resilience, rather than highlighting personal limitations. This program was well received by school staff, although they expressed barriers to implementation, including resistance from school administrators.[19] Subsequent trials of the program evidenced increases in self-efficacy and coping skills, however self-injury was not assessed in the trials.[20] Training of school staff in delivery of the program also appears to offer benefit and increase perceptions of the ability to deliver solution-focused approaches to mental health promotion in schools.[21] These preliminary findings suggest that a strengths-based approach to understanding and addressing self-injury will also have benefit, and will help alleviate the pitfalls often associated with medical or deficit-based models of care.

PERSON-CENTERED FRAMING OF SELF-INJURY

Central to a person-centered framing of self-injury is the recognition that the experience of self-injury will be different for every individual. This includes reasons someone started to self-injure, what maintains the behavior, experiences of being someone who self-injures (including consideration of stigma, scarring, navigating disclosures), and experiences related to self-injury recovery. While there may be some generalities, it is best not to make any assumptions about what an individual's personal experience is. For this reason, inclusion of individuals with lived experience is essential to fostering a person-centered approach to both research and clinical care.

An expert panel convened by the World Health Organization has offered practical guidelines for conducting patient-centered health research.[22] While individuals who self-injure may not always be considered patients, the same principles can be used to guide person-centered research practices in self-injury. These guidelines include:

- The perspective of the individual being critical in research and treatment guidelines
- Using multiple and complementary forms of engagement, matched to the issue and context being studied
- Transparency about the role of individuals with lived experience
- Broad representation and consideration of equity, diversity, and inclusive practice
- Including at least two individuals with lived experience throughout the research process
- Providing adequate information and support to the representatives
- Teaching researchers the knowledge and skills to support engagement with individuals with lived experience
- Allocate adequate resources in terms of time, money, and energy
- Continually monitor and measure interactions to allow refinement of procedures if needed
  (adapted from de Wit et al., 2019)

In clinical practice, person-centered approaches have long been championed throughout the health sector (see Chapter 14 for suggestions on how to approach advocacy in research, practice, and outreach efforts). Person (or patient) centered approaches advocate for inclusion of the patient in decisions about their treatment, rather than being treated as passive consumers. Here, researchers and clinicians emphasize the need to adopt a person-centered approach at three levels: the structural or organizational level, the process or patient–healthcare provider level, and the outcome or ongoing care level.[23,24] This approach is associated with social and physical well-being, and satisfaction with care among patients with multiple health needs.[25] We have similarly suggested that a person-centered approach will be related to improved outcomes for individuals who are discussing their self-injury with a healthcare professional[26,27] or in a school setting.[28,29]

CONCLUSION

In writing this book, we hope to challenge people's thinking about self-injury, with a focus on understanding the "experience" of self-injury, not just factors that may statistically increase or decrease risk of the behavior occurring. By adopting a person-centered approach, informed by voices of those with lived experience, we can start to understand what it is like for someone who self-injures and how they navigate the world around them. Traditional scientific research has taught us a lot about self-injury, but only by listening to individuals who have self-injured can we start to really understand why someone might self-injure, and what it means to them. Throughout this book we adopt a person-centered lens to better understand the stigma associated with self-injury (Chapter 4), outline appropriate language to use when talking about self-injury (Chapter 5), consider contagion and the impact of social media (Chapters 6 and 7), demonstrate how a person-centered approach can be applied in different contexts such as schools (Chapter 8) and families (Chapter 9), and how this approach can be used to conceptualize and make meaning of self-injury intervention (Chapter 10), recovery (Chapters 11 and 12), and supporting others who self-injure (Chapter 13).

Self-Injury and Stigma

Self-injury has been historically misunderstood. Unfortunately, despite many advances in what we know about it, self-injury also remains highly stigmatized.[1-4] However, recent efforts have yielded a new theoretical framework with which to understand this stigma. We therefore focus this chapter on the nature of this model. We then discuss the implications of this model along with potential avenues to address stigma as this area gains more research attention. Toward the end of the chapter, we draw attention to the centrality of a nonstigmatizing, person-centered approach when working with individuals with lived experience of self-injury.

UNDERSTANDING STIGMA

Prior to discussing self-injury stigma specifically, it is important to first provide a brief overview of stigma more generally. Stigma is the product of several factors but tends to begin with labeling and stereotyping.[5-7] First, an individual is identified due to a mark that is considered socially aberrant or unacceptable. This "mark" may be due to a particular behavior (e.g., drug use), condition (e.g., HIV), or physical attribute (e.g., body type). For instance, someone who has schizophrenia may be pejoratively labeled as *crazy* or as a *schizophrenic*. From here, stereotypes, which refer to ways that people organize information about different groups, are applied. In the case of stigma, these stereotypes are negative. For example, someone with schizophrenia may be viewed as dangerous and violent; someone with depression might be viewed as lazy and weak. Next, people must agree with the stereotype. When this happens, they tend to respond to the stereotype with negative emotions (e.g., disgust, hate, fear) and in turn, behave in ways that align with their belief system. The result of this is prejudice and discrimination. As an example, if someone viewed people with schizophrenia as dangerous and violent, they may develop a sense of fear toward these individuals and perhaps with people who have mental illness more broadly. Stemming from this emotional response (fear), people may subsequently make conscious effort to avoid someone with schizophrenia or even act aggressively toward them (e.g., bullying, being confrontational or demeaning).

SELF-INJURY STIGMA

A review of the literature points to a range of misconceptions about self-injury, including the view that self-injury is attention-seeking and manipulative,[8–11] that the behavior is circumscribed to young people or represents an adolescent fad,[12,13] and that only girls or young women self-injure.[8] Taken together, these (as well as other) views can propagate stereotypes and provoke discrimination and other invalidating reactions toward people with lived experience.[2,14] Concerningly, when this transpires, people who self-injure may internalize these stereotypes, which foments negative views about oneself and an unwillingness to reach out to others for support.[2,15] In turn, this can exacerbate people's feelings of isolation and feeling misunderstood.[4]

As depicted in Table 4.1 the stigmatization of self-injury is complex and stigma can take on numerous forms.[4] One such manifestation of stigma involves

Table 4.1. FORMS AND EXAMPLES OF SELF-INJURY STIGMA.

Form of Stigma	Examples
Public Stigma	• *People who self-injure are weak.* • *People who self-injure are freaks.* • *Only crazy people self-injure.* • *Individuals who self-injure are manipulative and attention-seeking.*
Enacted Stigma	• *Denying people analgesia prior to suturing injuries.* • *Firing someone from a job after discovering their self-injury.* • *Not hiring a qualified job candidate because they have self-injured.* • *Not admitting a student to graduate school after reading about their lived experience in a personal statement.*
Self-Stigma	• *I'm weak for having self-injured.* • *I don't deserve support or to be cared for because of my self-injury.* • *My self-injury experience is not legitimate.* • *There is something wrong with me for having self-injured.*
Anticipated Stigma	• *If I tell my mom I'm cutting she'll think I'm just attention-seeking.* • *If my boss finds out I self-injure I'll lose my job.* • *I'll be ostracized by my family if they knew I self-injured.* • *Because of my self-injury, I can't get too close to others. They'll never accept me.*
Vicarious Stigma	• *News media articles propagating myths about self-injury (e.g., self-injury is attention-seeking).* • *Overhearing people make jokes about self-injury (though not directed at that individual).* • *TV or media portrayals of people who self-injure as weak or defective.* • *Seeing negative comments about people who self-injure online.*

public stigma,[6] which pertains to the attitudes and beliefs that society has about individuals who self-injure (e.g., *people who self-injure are weak; individuals who self-injure are manipulative and attention-seeking*). Another form of stigma is enacted stigma,[16] which entails explicit discriminatory behaviors toward people who self-injure (e.g., *deciding to not hire an otherwise qualified person after seeing visible scarring from self-injury; not giving someone an anesthetic if their injuries need suturing*). These first two forms of stigma involve how others view or respond to people who self-injure. However, stigma can also be experienced within. That is, people may internalize public stigma in the form of self-stigma[6] (e.g., *I don't deserve support or help because I self-injure; I'm a weak person because of my self-injury*). Individuals with lived experience may also have anticipated stigma.[17] This occurs when individuals expect and worry that others will be stigmatizing toward them, irrespective of any prior interactions (e.g., *If I disclose that I self-injure, people will think I'm disgusting; If someone finds out I self-injure, they will shame me*). Finally, we recently suggested a fifth form of stigma—namely, vicarious stigma.[18] Specifically, we posit that this occurs when an individual is exposed to messages or content about self-injury that is not directed to them specifically but that still carries a stigmatizing undertone (e.g., seeing stigmatizing messages in the media, overhearing people joke about self-injury). Certainly, vicarious stigma is fueled by public stigma. However, the focus here is on the impact of continued exposure to these vicarious messages on people with lived experience. Notably, this can involve internalized stigma.

Over the years, there have been enumerable accounts of stigma toward people who self-injure, including in layperson,[1] healthcare,[19-21] and school settings.[22,23] In line with this, individuals who self-injure frequently report negative reactions from others which, in turn, brings about reluctance to disclose their self-injury in the future.[14,24] Indeed, many people who self-injure experience significant shame, embarrassment, and invalidation.[14,24,25] Unfortunately, these kinds of experiences can have numerous deleterious effects beyond their psychological impact. This includes thwarted help-seeking and hopelessness about the prospect of recovery.[2,26] When considering the seriousness of self-injury and the risks associated with repeated self-injury, including the risk for suicidal thinking and behavior discussed in Chapter 2, the impact of stigma is highly concerning.

In many ways, the above consequences of self-injury stigma mirror those reported in other areas in which stigma is well-documented (e.g., HIV, mental illness, disability).[27,28] Despite these parallels, the stigmatization of self-injury is ostensibly unique given the many considerations (e.g., its self-inflicted nature, scarring) that need to be taken into account.[4] Indeed, to work toward effective antistigma initiatives, having a conceptual framework to both understand and study self-injury stigma is needed. Thus, below, we present a newly offered framework with which to conceptualize self-injury stigma.[4]

SELF-INJURY STIGMA FRAMEWORK

Informed by prior stigma work[6,17,28] the self-injury stigma framework offers a model to situate and understand the stigmatization of self-injury (see Figure 4.1). This involves six key domains that are thought to underpin self-injury stigma (i.e., what about self-injury may contribute to stigma), namely: origin, concealability, course, peril, disruptiveness, and aesthetics. Although these are clearly demarcated on the following pages, it is important to bear in mind that different model components may have simultaneous relevance.

Origin

The first part of the model involves origin, which has to do with the onset of self-injury and the corresponding views that people hold about why individuals self-injure. In particular, origin involves the manner by which people are blamed for having engaged in self-injury—they are blamed as they are considered responsible for engaging in it. Indeed, if someone is rendered responsible for a given behavior or condition, they are apt to be blamed for it.[28] In line with this, past work on stigma has illustrated that conditions that one acquires (e.g., HIV contracted

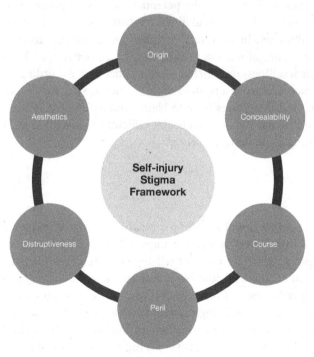

Figure 4.1. Self-injury stigma framework.

through unsafe sexual practices) engender more stigma than those that are not (e.g., being born with a particular physical health condition).[29] This is due to the view that a person could have made efforts to prevent or avoid the onset of the acquired mark, also referred to as an onset-attribution. In this way, because self-injury is seen to be under the volitional control of the person who self-injures, it elicits more stigma. For example, an individual who self-injures may be blamed for having self-injured, and thus seen as attention-seeking. When this occurs, it may result in them being discriminated against (e.g., not being offered mental health or medical services) or experiencing negative reactions from other people (e.g., being yelled at or demeaned). Therefore, without an appreciation and understanding for why people may self-injure, reactions such as these are more apt to occur.

Concealability

The second part of the model is concealability, which has to do with self-injury's visibility to others—including both the injuries resulting from the behavior and the potential for permanent scarring. According to theory, the greater the degree of visibility a marking has (e.g., minor versus extensive scarring), the more stigmatized it may be.[28] This stigma is, in turn, exacerbated by the blame that people who self-injure may receive if they are viewed as responsible for their own scarring. Compounding this is the potential for concealability to also implicate the stigma associated with mental illness.[4] When compared to most other mental health difficulties, self-injury is not "invisible" and is thus not always concealable. Hence, the presence of self-injury scars may be an outward indicator of the existence of mental illness or a mental health difficulty.[30] Accordingly, people who self-injure may experience a twofold stigma—they are stigmatized for having deliberately injured themselves (due to blame and being held responsible for the behavior) and for having a mental health difficulty or mental illness (due to self-injury signaling its potential presence).

Course

The course domain within the model pertains to the temporal nature of self-injury; that is, how self-injury engagement changes with time.[28] Inasmuch as people may be held responsible for the onset of self-injury as described earlier, people may also be blamed and held responsible if they are viewed as being in control of the *offset* of their condition.[31] Thus, a person could be deemed responsible for their self-injury and subsequently stigmatized if they are not taking active steps to stop self-injuring—also referred to as an offset attribution. Clearly, stopping self-injury is much easier said than done. Recovery is highly complex and represents an ongoing, nonlinear process.[32,33] Self-injury recovery does not occur right away. If it were truly that easy, people would simply stop. While a fulsome discussion of recovery is presented in Chapter 11, misunderstandings about recovery (e.g., that it is, or should be, easy to stop) may nonetheless play a role in the stigmatization of self-injury.

At the same time, it is important to keep in mind that just because one has stopped self-injury and is viewed as having recovered does not mean that they are immune to stigma.[4] As mentioned before, the residual scarring from self-injury can provoke stigma;[1,4,34] in this way, people may encounter stigma if they choose to disclose their experience and are responded to inappropriately. Therefore, the issue of stigma may have ongoing temporal relevance for individuals with lived experience and it should not be assumed that when someone no longer self-injures that stigma ceases to be a concern.

Peril

The aspect of peril within the model involves the extent to which a mark signals danger. The greater the danger associated with a mark (i.e., the more peril), the more stigma it will have.[28] Yet, there is a dichotomy with regard to peril in the context of self-injury.[4] On the one hand, self-injury may be viewed as intrinsically linked to suicide and, as such, perilous. This is unsurprising given their historical conflation. Along these lines, people may self-injure in ways that yield injuries that are more medically severe than intended; and, in rare cases, individuals may injure themselves in ways that result in accidental death. In these (and other) instances, self-injury would be rendered perilous due to its high degree of perceived danger.[4] On the other hand, self-injury may also be dismissed as trivial or in simplistic and reductionist manners (e.g., assuming self-injury is teenage fad).[4] Should this occur, it may be viewed as a behavior not warranting much of a response. Although the trivialization of self-injury may, at first, seem to contradict how peril is conceptualized in the framework, dismissive and trivializing reactions nonetheless indicate stigma. Indeed, there are numerous reports that self-injury may be dismissed as a legitimate concern, including in healthcare settings, which can result in poor treatment experiences.[14,35]

Aesthetics

The next component of the model, aesthetics, involves how visibly displeasing a given mark may be. Specifically, there is a tendency for people to liken attractiveness with morality. Thus, people who are seen as unattractive would also be seen as immoral.[28] Applied to self-injury, the visible and perceived displeasing nature of injuries or scarring could result in stigma. Correspondingly, the more visible or extensive one's injuries or scarring may be, the more stigma one would likely experience. Consistent with this, there are many reports from people who engage in self-injury that others have viewed their scars as "gross" or "ugly" and that self-injury, itself, is viewed as a "disgusting" behavior.[14,36] Not only do these reports signal the presence of outward stigma, but they can also be internalized by people with lived experience, which can bring about shame, marginalization, and isolation.[15,34,37] To this end, and understandably, some individuals will go to great lengths to conceal their self-injury from others.

Disruptiveness

Finally, disruptiveness pertains to how a mark impacts or interferes with one's relationships. The more interference, the greater the potential for stigma.[28] In the context of self-injury, this will vary considerably on the basis of the context and the type of a person's relationship with others. In many instances, self-injury can be concealed and thus the impact on relationships would be minimal (e.g., someone hiding scars from a coworker). In others, however, this may not be feasible. For example, in the case of intimate, romantic relationships, it is likely much more difficult to conceal self-injury; likewise, concealing self-injury may prove difficult in the summer months when people are more likely to wear short sleeves or shorts. As a result, people with lived experience of self-injury may have significant trepidation about being in particular environments or developing relationships altogether.

Disruption also has relevance when considering how people respond to individuals who have self-injured. Unsurprisingly, these reactions are—for many people—highly salient. They can influence the likelihood of future disclosures as well as impact the nature of an existing relationship. If someone responds poorly to a disclosure of self-injury, this may jeopardize the quality (and perhaps the duration) of that relationship. Should this happen, it may leave the person who self-injures feeling alone and invalidated. At the same time, if the response was appropriate, it might strengthen the relationship while providing the individual who self-injures validation and acceptance. For these reasons, the response to disclosures and how people interact with individuals with lived experience regarding self-injury is critical. We address a person-centered approach to interacting with people who engage in self-injury in Chapter 13.

IMPLICATIONS AND FUTURE DIRECTIONS

Until now, there has not been a conceptual framework for use in the understanding of self-injury stigma. In this regard, the self-injury stigma framework[4] offers a useful heuristic to inform research that not only works to understand the nature and impact of self-injury stigma but also highlights how such stigma transpires. By virtue of elucidating what may underlie and drive self-injury stigma, more focused efforts can be put in place to combat it. Indeed, each of the relevant domains of the model has relevance to the manners by which stigma manifests outlined earlier, namely: public, self, enacted, anticipated, and vicarious stigma. Table 4.2 therefore presents an overview of the model and its application to these forms of stigma. With this in mind, we now turn to a discussion

Table 4.2 OVERVIEW AND APPLICATION OF THE SELF-INJURY STIGMA FRAMEWORK TO DIFFERENT FORMS OF STIGMA.

Self-injury Stigma Framework Domain	Type of Stigma				
	Public	Self	Anticipated	Enacted	Vicarious
Origin	Reading a magazine article that says the "Internet is creating a cult of self-injures."	"There is something deeply wrong with me for having self-injured."	"People will think I'm crazy if they find out I self-injure."	A doctor saying: "You seem like a bright person, why are you doing something [self-injury] so irrational?"	Overhearing a conversation on the bus in which someone who self-injures is called "unhinged."
Concealability	An employment setting mandating the covering of all scarring related to self-injury.	"I can't stand my scars so need to hide them from the world."	"If I wear shirtsleeves at the party everyone will see that I used to self-injure."	Being at a grocery store and someone coming up to a person to say "what were you thinking doing that to your arms?"	Watching a show in which a character says: "They're only flaunting their scars to get notices."
Course	Someone who believes "people who self-injure should just be able to stop."	"Recovery is impossible so why bother trying?"	"My mom will think I'll be self-injuring forever."	A nurse telling someone in the emergency room that "self-injury is a phase that you should just get over"	Hearing a teacher talk about self-injury as a "superficial fad that teens just to through."
Peril	People thinking that self-injury is simply a 'feigned suicide attempt.'	"I can't work as a counsellor, I'm just not safe to be around"	"My clients will think I'm suicidal and take their business away if they find out about my self-injury"	A friend rolling their eyes and saying "Geesh . . . why not just get it right and end it all now?"	Seeing trolling comments online that 'cutters should stop now and end their lives'
Aesthetics	Reading an editorial in which the author refers to people who 'destroy their bodies' through self-injury.	"My body is ruined because I self-injured."	"If my partner and I are intimate they'll think I'm gross with all these scars"	A swimming coach telling a team member: "you won't make it to the next level with those scars."	Observing an employer telling a co-worker: "Please roll down your sleeves so you don't scare away business."
Disruptiveness	Being a student in a school that has a policy for a "self-injury contagion"	"I'll be alone forever because of my self-injury."	"If my older sister finds out she'll think I'm a manipulative attention-seeker."	Being told by a faculty mentor that one shouldn't pursue a career as a therapist because of their self-injury.	Hearing that a coach noticed a teammate's self-injury and said: "what a pointless thing to do to yourself"

about how this model has promise to be meaningfully applied to advance research as well as address stigma.

Research Implications: Framework Utility and Sources of Stigma

A natural first step for researchers is to establish an evidence base for the model's utility. Insight into the many paths to stigma would help to outline different ways to address and reduce stigma. Certainly, as discussed throughout this chapter, there are bound to be many sources of stigma. One such consideration though is the role that media plays. Indeed, news media has been implicated as playing a role in the communication and perpetuation of stereotypes more broadly,[38] including representing a source of stereotypes and misrepresentations of mental illness.[39,40] Also important is examining the role that the Internet and social media play in the propagation of self-injury stigma. The Internet and social media may have relevance for a few reasons. First, many people across the globe obtain news via social media; this may be another avenue by which news media is accessed. Thus, if news media share stories with stigmatizing content, there is a good likelihood these stories are accessed via social media. Second, prior research has established that myths about self-injury are common on health websites,[8] and that people may be exposed to stigmatizing content when communicating online. In this regard, given the salience of the Internet as a medium for people who self-injure to connect with and support one another,[8] stigma propagation on social media should be explored more fully. Finally, social media is constantly changing and, as such, it will be important for researchers to keep up-to-speed regarding how new online platforms could play a role in fomenting stigma.

While these endeavors represent just some of the ways that sources of self-injury stigma can be explored, the significance of these efforts is noteworthy. Indeed, by virtue of undertaking such initiatives, researchers will be well positioned to not only determine when and where stigma is present but to identify what aspects of the self-injury stigma framework may have relevance. For example, if media stories emphasize the need to ban self-injury content online, this may inform the public's perceptions of concealability and aesthetics. From here, this might shape stereotypes about self-injury, thereby eliciting public stigma as well as exacerbating self and anticipated stigma among individuals with lived experience. A natural next step in this line of inquiry is to ascertain whether and how media-rooted stereotypes engender negative attitudes in society. This would allow for a greater understanding of the kinds of beliefs that people have, how pervasive they are, and what domains in the model seem to be most relevant. Knowing which domains are most salient would, in turn, help to focus where antistigma efforts are most needed.

Research Implications: Relevance to Lived Experience

As people with lived experience are self-injury experts in their own right,[41] working to develop a deeper understanding of their experiences with stigma, including its impact is essential. This can involve working with individuals to ascertain what they see as contributing to self-injury stigma and, as such, which domains comprising the self-injury stigma framework have relevance in their experience. Alongside these efforts, it will be important to explore which stigma-related constructs are most relevant to their experience, including self, enacted, anticipated, and vicarious stigma. From here, understanding how these manifestations of stigma impact people's lives would be important (e.g., on disclosure, in the context of recovery).

To optimally address these lines of research, it will be important to not just involve people with lived experience as participants in research but to seek their insight in terms of how approaches to research can be enhanced. Hence, individuals with lived experience ought to play an active role throughout the research process.[41,42] For example, involving people in the context of focus groups may help to determine the kinds of questions to ask of participants in future studies. As another example, researchers could establish advisory boards or hold panels at academic meetings that involve lived experience perspectives. Doing so would help to ensure a more priority-driven research agenda when it comes to better understanding self-injury stigma, and as discussed, later, how to ideally address it.

Measuring Self-Injury Stigma

Historically, efforts to measure stigma in the context of self-injury have relied on scales that tap into attitudes toward behaviors related to self-injury (e.g., deliberate self-harm)[43] or those that are adapted from measures that pertain to the stigma associated with mental illness.[44,45] In the case of the latter, researchers have had to modify the wording of scales to ask about self-injury specifically. Arguably, these efforts are limited as they are broader in nature, may carry assumptions (i.e., that a question about mental illness stigma has direct applicability to self-injury), and they do not map onto the theoretical framework for self-injury discussed earlier. For these reasons, we have recently been involved in the development of a measure specific to self-injury stigma that is informed by the model presented earlier.[46] Preliminary findings indicate that the measure has promising factorial validity and internal consistency. Moving forward, it will be important to use the measure among different populations and in various contexts. Nevertheless, this newly developed scale addresses an important gap in the field and has promise to offer a valid and reliable means of assessing the multi-faceted nature of self-injury stigma.

Addressing Self-Injury Stigma

Finally, and perhaps most importantly, antistigma initiatives are needed. This will no doubt require time and a multipronged approach. Although there are clearly several considerations to address in order to meaningfully inform antistigma efforts, it may be fruitful to draw from existing approaches used to address stigma in other areas and tailor these to the context of self-injury. In doing so, it will be important to ensure that these efforts attend to the unique factors that play a role in the context of self-injury stigma.

Certainly, one part of any agenda to tackle self-injury stigma will involve enhancing self-injury literacy and debunking existing stereotypes. However, provision of accurate information—on its own—will likely be insufficient. Instead, involvement of people with lived experience will be vital to the success of antistigma efforts. Supporting this is both evidence and calls from leading researchers involved in antistigma work in the area of mental illness, who underscore the significance of directly involving people with lived experience in antistigma work.[2,47-49] Notably, Corrigan calls for antistigma efforts that involve contact sessions in which people hear directly from individuals with lived experience.[6] Importantly, contact-based initiatives have demonstrated more effectiveness when compared to traditional approaches that emphasize just knowledge provision.[5,49] For these reasons, researchers have similarly called for the use of these approaches and broader participatory-based approaches to address the stigmatization of self-injury.[41,42]

SUMMARY

As should now be clear, self-injury stigma is both complex and multifaceted in nature. Such stigma can also deeply impact people with lived experience. Indeed, there are numerous proximal (e.g., invalidation, shame) and distal (e.g., reluctance to seek further support, thwarted recovery efforts and continued self-injury) consequences of self-injury stigma.[4] For these reasons it is essential that a nonstigmatizing approach be used in myriad contexts, including but not limited to: how we talk (and write) about self-injury (including the language we use); how we study self-injury (i.e., how research is conducted); and how we address self-injury in different settings such as schools and clinical contexts (e.g., assessment, intervention). In the absence of such an approach, individuals may be left feeling misunderstood and marginalized. For these reasons, the person-centered framework outlined in the previous chapter is integrated throughout our book's subsequent chapters.

Use of Appropriate Language to Discuss Self-Injury

WHY IS LANGUAGE IMPORTANT?

Spoken and written language not only provide modes of communication but also help shape attitudes and how the world is viewed. Language is used to share ideas, voice opinions, convey thoughts and feelings, and create a common understanding. Importantly, words are used to convey meaning, but this meaning can go beyond the strict dictionary definition of a word. Meanings are socially constructed; they take shape through interaction with others and the world around us.[1] As such, meanings, and the way language is used, can change over time. Take the word "gay" for example. Originally used to mean carefree or cheerful, today the word refers to someone who identifies as homosexual. Even in that context, the word takes on different meanings; while LGBTIQ+ groups advocate use of the word "gay" to identify men who are attracted to other men, the term can also be used in a pejorative sense (e.g., "that's so gay" as an insult). Effective communication requires that the people communicating apply the same meaning to the words being used. In applying meaning to words, we must also be mindful of the impact words can have on societal attitudes and on individuals. The old adage "sticks and stones can break my bones, but words can never harm me" simply is not true. Words are powerful, as any speechwriter would attest. While they can be more effective in conflict resolution than physical aggression (i.e., "the pen is mightier than the sword") they can also cause lasting damage to an individual's self-worth if used in a pejorative or stigmatizing way.

In recognition of the potential for language to foster stigma, there has been a relatively long history of adopting person-centered language within psychiatric and mental health discourse. Rather than labeling and pathologizing, mental health professionals are urged to use "person-first" language rather than "disorder-first" language.[2] Other fields have been slower to adopt person-centered language. Despite widespread media guidelines for reporting on mental illness, media reports frequently contain sensationalist and stigmatizing language[3] (see Chapter 4). In Canada, a case file review of judges' decisions involving people with mental illness revealed that although most judges used respectful language, there were notable instances in which stigmatizing language was used.[4] For example, judges noted plaintiffs' failure to *admit* to their mental illness, implying mental illness is something to be hidden, and "confessed." They also made mention of people being *arrested* under the Mental Health Act, despite often being aware that being apprehended under the Act is not an arrest. Examples of use of archaic terms such as "insane" and "lunatic" were also noted, and disorder-first language (e.g., "schizophrenic") was common.

As noted in Chapter 4, self-injury carries significant stigma that can be internalized by individuals who self-injure. Use of pejorative, or stigmatizing, language can lead to individuals who self-injure feeling further misunderstood, and leads to society "othering" individuals who self-injure. This "othering" creates the sense that people who self-injure are somehow different from people who do not self-injure, and deserve to be treated differently. Such public stigma can then be internalized by the individual, such that they believe they are different from others (e.g., crazy), and deserve to be treated differently (e.g., not deserving of help). In this way, the resultant self-stigma can foster feelings of shame and guilt, and lead individuals to stay silent about their self-injury. Fear of anticipated stigma, how people will react to disclosure, in turn, reduces support-seeking behavior, even if an individual believes they would benefit from support.[5] It is important then that people are mindful of the language used when talking about self-injury, and individuals with lived experience of self-injury, so as to avoid further stigma.

HOW DOES LANGUAGE SHAPE ATTITUDES?

According to social identity theory, we base our sense of identity on the groups to which we assign ourselves.[6] The first step in this identity formation is to categorize people into groups, and to place ourselves in a group. Naturally, we can belong to multiple groups (e.g., based on gender, age, sporting team supported). Next, is to begin to identify with the characteristics of this group, and act in ways that are consistent with the characteristics of the group. For example, if someone categorizes themselves as a football fan, they might attend football games, purchase their team's merchandise, and become upset when the team loses. Finally, we engage in social comparison, comparing our group to other groups. This could be either an upward social comparison (comparing our group to groups we think are better than ours) or downward social comparison[7] (comparing our group to groups we think are inferior). Thus, individuals form in-groups (our group) and out-groups (groups we do not belong to). A key tenet of social identity theory is that people will look for negative characteristics of the out-group, in order to enhance the image of the in-group. At its extreme, division of the in-group and out-group can lead to racism, sexism, prejudice, and discrimination. In the context of self-injury, the same process can be used to categorize people who self-injure into an out-group, and to assign stigmatized characteristics to this group.

One of the ways in-group identity is strengthened, and the distance from the out-group is enhanced, is through targeted use of language. For example, football fans have been demonstrated to use a linguistic pattern of irony as a form of aggression when commenting on behaviors of rival football teams, whereas literal comments are used when talking about their own team's performance.[8] In general, people tend to use abstract language to describe positive in-group behaviors and negative out-group behaviors, and more concrete language to describe negative in-group and positive out-group behaviors.[9] Importantly, people can identify which group others belong to based on the kind of language they use, even if these are only subtle linguistic differences.[10] Linguistic framing can also influence judgments people make. In one study, the use of agentic language in a vignette about a fire being started at a restaurant table ("She had ignited the napkin" vs. "The napkin had ignited"), resulted in participants ascribing more blame to the individual and recommending increased payment for the damage.[11]

As applied to self-injury, use of pejorative or stigmatizing language further distances individuals who self-injure from the in-group—categorizing them as inferior to people who do not self-injure. Individuals who self-injure are then likely to be viewed as a homogeneous group, with common identifying characteristics and behaviors. Picking up on this linguistic intergroup bias, individuals who self-injure are likely to see themselves as belonging to the out-group, and feeling that others do not understand them. A person-centered approach to self-injury requires that we reduce this in-group out-group comparison, and instead focus on the experiences of the individual person.

According to communication theories, the likelihood that language will change attitudes depends on how credible the source is.[12] This credibility is determined by how confidently and articulately the speaker communicates and the normative expectations held by the listener. If the message content conforms to social norms, the listener is more likely to accept the message and change their attitudes accordingly. Importantly, the act of describing the topic of interest (i.e., self-injury) can reinforce the communicator's own attitudes. Given that news media is a trusted source of information,[13] the potential for messages conveyed by the media may be particularly persuasive. Similarly, clinicians and researchers considered experts in the field are also likely to promote negative attitudes and stigma if they use pejorative or stigmatizing language.

THE MEDICALIZATION OF SELF-INJURY

While there have been moves to depathologize or demedicalize mental illness, it seems the opposite is true of self-injury. Over time, self-injury has become more prominent in psychological and psychiatric discourses, perhaps reflecting greater awareness of the behavior. Inclusion of the proposed Non-Suicidal Self-Injury Disorder in the *Diagnostic and Statistical Manual of Mental Disorders* (DSM, 5th ed.[14]), as a condition warranting further investigation, seems to cement its place in the medical field. However, this medicalization of self-injury neglects the fact that self-injury is a *behavior*. It is not a disease or a disorder, but a coping strategy people use to manage intense or unwanted emotions. From this perspective it does not make a lot of sense to consider self-injury from a medical viewpoint.[15] Even within the proposed DSM criteria for Non-Suicidal Self-Injury Disorder, the primary criteria are engagement in the behavior, to alter an emotional or interpersonal state. That is, there is not a core set of symptoms that might characterize a disorder.

Yet, disease discourse is common when discussing self-injury. Perhaps the most obvious example of this is in discussions of self-injury contagion. This language is borrowed from the area of infectious diseases, with the suggestion that self-injury can simply spread from person to person like an infectious disease.[15] This is not only untrue (see Chapter 6 for a detailed discussion of socialization effects), but implies individuals who self-injure are unwell or sick in some way. Individuals who have a contagious disease are usually asked to keep away from other people until they are well. This approach has also been taken with individuals who self-injure, with some schools demanding that students remain at home until injuries heal.[16]

The notion of contagion is also associated with fear; we typically avoid anything that might be contagious. It is perhaps not surprising then, that schools, mental health professionals, and medical staff in hospitals or psychiatric units sometimes fear discussing self-injury, not only due their own discomfort with the behavior, but out of concern for other students or patients who might "catch" self-injury.[16,17] However, rather than protecting students and patients, this unwillingness to discuss self-injury further silences individuals who self-injure, and keeps them very much in the out-group.

Another example of language being used to medicalize self-injury is in discussion of the course of self-injury. Clinicians and researchers refer to *recovery* from self-injury, and describe set-backs as a *relapse*. Recovery again implies that there is something to recover from, yet self-injury is usually the symptom of an underling concern, not the condition that needs to be treated.[15] Some do argue that, over time, repeated self-injury may become the primary concern, or that self-injury should be stopped before any underlying concern is addressed.[18] However, remember that self-injury is a behavior individuals use to help them cope, and we do not usually talk about recovering from coping strategies. Further, recovery is defined as a "return to a *normal* state of health, mind, or strength,"[19] which implies that an individual who self-injures is not normal. Continued use of such language can further promote stigma and lowered self-worth for individuals who self-injure, particularly those who experience ongoing thoughts about self-injury long after engaging in the behavior. We do use the term "recovery" in this book, and it is a term many with lived experience use to describe their experiences; however we hope that we have assigned a different meaning to the word. Specifically we view recovery as much more than simply cessation of self-injury, and as a concept that will mean different things to different people (see Chapter 11 for a new conceptualization of recovery).

The notion of relapse is one borrowed from the alcohol and other drug field, where someone who has abstained for some time, begins to drink or use drugs again. The same approach is applied to self-injury, where someone who engages in self-injury after a long period of not engaging in it is considered to have relapsed. The terminology here is problematic for a number of reasons. First is the association with addictive behaviors. Although self-injury has been likened to addictive behaviors,[20] and some individuals with lived experience describe it as an addiction,[21] there are many features that differentiate self-injury and addictive behaviors.[22] Situating self-injury in the addiction space risks removing autonomy from the individual, and does not address the reasons someone self-injures or the function it serves for them. Second, recovery is not a linear process.[23,24] Set-backs are bound to happen, and the negative connotations associated with relapse may lead an individual to feel like a failure for engaging in self-injury. Finally, when framed in the context of relapse, these set-backs may foster hopelessness for the future, and a lack of confidence in the recovery process. We propose that instead of labeling any set-backs as relapse, that individuals normalize ongoing thoughts and urges to self-injure, and recognize that recovery is not a linear, straightforward process.

Another way we see language used to medicalize self-injury is in describing the behavior as maladaptive[25] (e.g., a maladaptive coping strategy). While not necessarily borrowed from the medical lexicon directly, the word maladaptive conjures images that something is wrong with the person. While it is usually the behavior, and not the person, that is described as maladaptive, as noted above individuals can internalize language and assign the same meaning to themselves. Thus, someone who engages in a behavior that is labeled as maladaptive may come to view themselves as maladaptive. Further, use of the term maladaptive implies that self-injury is not effective as a coping strategy, and ignores the experience of individuals who find self-injury to be an effective means of emotion regulation. This invalidation of the individual's experience is counter to the person-centered approach we advocate.

PERSON-CENTERED LANGUAGE

In contrast to the medicalized terms described above (contagion, relapse, maladaptive), and in line with movements in the broader mental health field, we advocate use of person-centered language to talk about self-injury and individuals who self-injure (see Table 5.1). This means focusing on the individual, and not on their history of self-injury and avoiding reductionist terms such as "self-injurer" and "cutter" which define people by the behavior.[26] Since the inclusion of Non-Suicidal Self-Injury Disorder in the DSM, as a condition warranting further study, there has been a shift toward talking about people "with self-injury." While this is no doubt an effort to use person-centered language, as we would talk about people with schizophrenia (rather than as schizophrenic), self-injury is still a behavior

Table 5.1. APPROPRIATE LANGUAGE TO USE WHEN TALKING ABOUT SELF-INJURY.

Most Appropriate Terminology	Least Appropriate Terminology
• Someone with lived experience	• Attention seeking
• Someone with a history of NSSI	• Hopeless
• Recovery from NSSI	• Manipulative
• Urges to self-injure	• Borderline
• Coping phrases	• Unstable personality
• Ongoing NSSI	• Cutter
• Recurrence of NSSI	• Person struggling to cope
	• Self-injurer
	• Contagion

not a disorder. As such, this phrasing does not make grammatical sense; it would be akin to talking about someone "with drinking" rather than someone with an alcohol use disorder.

In a recent study,[27] we invited clinicians and researchers to share the terms they use when talking about self-injury and compared their usage with terms and phrases they considered to be appropriate to use. We also invited people with lived experience to indicate the terms they considered most appropriate. Encouragingly, researchers and clinicians did not tend to use the phrases they considered most inappropriate (e.g., "manipulative," "attention seeking"), but they underused phrases that people with lived experience considered most appropriate to use ("people with a history of self-injury," "people with lived experience of self-injury"). This disconnect between language used by clinicians and researchers and that considered appropriate by individuals with lived self-injury experience highlights the need to include people with lived experience in conversations about self-injury, conversations about what is appropriate when talking about self-injury more broadly, and the impact that language use has on them.

CONCLUSION

Language is a powerful form of communication that can shape how we view the world, and how we interact with it. Language can foster negative attitudes and stigma, and can negatively impact people on the receiving end of pejorative or stigmatizing words. However, language can also educate, unite, and validate individuals. With this in mind, we call on all researchers and clinicians to reflect on the language they use to talk about self-injury, and consider the impact this may have on individuals with lived self-injury experience.

Rethinking and Addressing Contagion

As outlined in the previous chapter, the term "contagion" is problematic for a number of reasons. This includes the medicalization of self-injury, the potential to foster stigma, and the inherent fear that the term conjures. This fear then precludes talking about self-injury and results in excessive anxiety for individuals, families, healthcare professionals, and schools. For this reason, we avoid use of the word "contagion" in this chapter. Instead we talk about selection effects (where like-minded individuals tend to form peer groups with similar traits or interests), socialization effects (where knowing someone who self-injures increases risk of subsequent occurrences of self-injury), and peer influences to refer to a broader category of peer effects.

THE RELATION BETWEEN PEER EXPOSURE AND SELF-INJURY

One of the most consistent findings across the literature is that people who self-injure tend to know other people who self-injure. This holds among adolescents,[1-3] university students,[4-6] and clinical samples.[2] It also seems the more people an individual knows to self-injure, the more likely they are to self-injure.[4,7] However, it is difficult to tease out selection effects from socialization effects. That is, it is often not known if like-minded peers are attracted to each other and select peer groups who are similar to them (including in a history of self-injury), or whether socialization processes occur, whereby an individual gains the idea to self-injure from peers.[8,9]

In an inpatient sample, Prinstein and colleagues noted that adolescents' self-injury was associated with perceptions of their peers' depressive symptoms, suggesting an underlying core similarity in psychological concerns rather than socialization of self-injury per se.[2] Support for socialization effects has also been found, among young people in particular, reporting that they gained the idea to self-injure from friends.[5,10] Among Chinese adolescents, You and colleagues[11] found support for both socialization and selection effects. Having a friend who self-injures was associated with subsequent self-injury, but adolescents also tended to join peer groups whose members already engaged in self-injury. Similarly, Prinstein[2] observed socialization effects among school-based adolescents, and evidence for both selection and socialization effects among adolescent inpatients.

Few researchers attempt to explore factors that may explain the relation between peer exposure and one's own self-injury. When they do, researchers typically find that the association is not straightforward, but is moderated by other variables. For example, in a longitudinal study with adolescents, we observed that there was only a relation between knowing someone else who self-injures and one's own later probability of self-injury for students reporting a significant number of negative life events.[1] There was no relation at all for students reporting few averse life events. Similarly, a friend's self-injury is only predictive of adolescents' later self-injury for those with greater difficulties regulating emotion.[3] It may also be that these socialization effects only hold for younger adolescents or only hold for girls.[2] More work is needed to determine who is most susceptible to peer influences, and who may be at greater risk of self-injury when exposed to the behavior.

MEDIA (AND SOCIAL MEDIA) EXPOSURE AND SELF-INJURY

Another area of concern is the potential for individuals to gain the idea to self-injure from media or social media, and an association between frequency of media exposure and frequency of self-injury has been noted.[12] In the suicide field, the potential for media publicity of high-profile suicides to increase risk of suicide among viewers is well noted.[13] For this reason, many countries have strict media reporting guidelines for suicide. These caution journalists to: avoid explicit mention of means of suicide, avoid stigmatizing language, use person-centered language when talking about suicide (see Chapter 2), and provide mental health resources with the article.[14] In Australia and the United Kingdom, guidelines are also provided for reporting of self-harm (broadly defined). Unfortunately, few news outlets appear to adhere to such guidelines. We conducted a content analysis[15] of news reporting of self-injury across Australia, New Zealand, Canada, the United States of America, and the United Kingdom. Approximately 40% of articles used a sensational headline, and one in five used stigmatizing language to describe self-injury. Two-thirds of articles explicitly reported method of self-injury. Although there is little work on how media reporting might increase rates of self-injury among readers, following patterns in the suicide literature, this sensationalized reporting, including detailed description of self-injury methods, is likely to prompt subsequent self-injurious behaviors. Media guidelines have only recently been developed for the appropriate reporting of self-injury.[16] These mirror the suicide reporting guidelines and emphasize the need for accurate and neutral information about self-injury, with a focus on stories of recovery and efforts to seek treatment.

Individuals also report gaining the idea to self-injure from television or movies.[17] Individuals are more likely to model behaviors exhibited by people they admire, where the consequences are seen as advantageous, and when they are exposed to multiple instances of the behavior.[18] In one of our studies, we noted that film depictions of self-injury tend to be sensationalized and feature self-injury prominently.[19] Self-injury was often associated with suicidal behavior, and few characters were receiving professional support at the time of the self-injury. In a follow-up study, the number of movies seen was associated with self-injury, particularly for participants who reported a decreased belief in their ability to resist urges to self-injure.[4] Similar to the effects noted for knowing peers who self-injure, it is unclear whether this association is due to selection or socialization effects. In our study, most participants reported that they were older when they saw the films than they were when they first self-injured, suggesting that people who self-injure are attracted to films that portray self-injury, rather than the films prompting the idea to self-injure.

Over the last decade, there has been concern that depictions of self-injury online and in social media may encourage self-injury. The effect of social media on self-injury is detailed in the following chapter so we will not dwell on it here. However, it is important to note that social media can have both beneficial and detrimental effects.[20] Concerns over the potential for social media to lead to self-injury and suicidal behavior have caused Facebook and Instagram to change their policies about posts related to self-injury. While they allow self-injury-related content, they remove content that encourages self-injury, as well as graphic images and real-time depictions that may be triggering or encourage others to engage in the behavior. These decisions have been made in consultation with experts in self-injury and suicidal behavior, who are cognizant of the potential for socialization effects associated with these behaviors. However, it is important to acknowledge that sharing experiences of self-injury can give individuals who self-injure a voice, foster a sense of belonging, and garner encouragement and support from others that may aid recovery.[20]

WHY DO SOCIALIZATION EFFECTS OCCUR?

One of the reported functions of self-injury is to bond with peers. Among university students, Heath and her colleagues[5] found that although emotional reasons for engaging in self-injury were most common, social motivations were reported by 65.2% of the sample. A large proportion of the sample reported talking about self-injury with their friends, and 4.3% had engaged in self-injury as a group. Among adolescents, individuals engaging in more severe self-injury are more likely to report self-injuring to belong to a group.[21] It is important to bear in mind that social support and a sense of belonging are also protective against self-injury. It may be that young people are talking to their friends about self-injury as a way of seeking support, not in a way that encourages or reinforces self-injury.

In a small number of studies, higher rates of self-injury have been noted among "alternative" subcultures such as Goth and emo groups.[22] In a German sample, Young and his colleagues[23] noted that adolescents self-identifying as belonging to an alternative subculture were more likely, than those who did not, to endorse both interpersonal and intrapersonal reasons for self-injury. Of note, they were more likely to endorse: "to feel more part of a group" and "to avoid being with people." Muehlenkamp and her colleagues[6] noted that social reasons for self-injury (e.g., wanting to fit in with others) were more often related to the initiation of self-injury, while emotion regulation reasons (e.g., cope with uncomfortable feelings) were related to repeated self-injury, with only 1.6% of the sample endorsing "to be part of a group" as a reason for ongoing self-injury.

Although these findings suggest some individuals may start to self-injure to feel a connection with peers, we cannot conclude that this reflects socialization effects. Of note, we do not know whether these individuals have gained the idea to self-injure from peers, or whether like-minded peers are attracted to each other, resulting in selection effects. Further, although some endorse social reasons for engaging in self-injury, this is rated as the least effective function of self-injury.

People endorsing social or interpersonal functions of self-injury are also likely to endorse intrapersonal functions, suggesting peer bonding is rarely the primary reason for self-injury.[24] In one study, individuals' therapists rated interpersonal reasons for self-injury as more relevant than the clients did.[25] Similar results were obtained with a college sample, with students with no history of self-injury viewing interpersonal reasons as more relevant than students with a history of self-injury.[26,27] These findings may reflect an overestimation, by individuals without lived self-injury experience, of the extent to which self-injury is motivated by affiliation with peer groups.

HOW DO SOCIALIZATION EFFECTS OCCUR?

Although individuals may self-injure to conform with peer expectations, or establish peer bonds, the primary reason people self-injure is to manage intense or unwanted emotions. So how do people learn that self-injury will be effective in doing this? In the 1970s Albert Bandura[18] proposed social learning theory to explain how children learn behaviors by imitating others. He suggested that children pay attention to the actions of other people around them, and subsequently model these behaviors. A key element of social learning theory was that people do not need to personally experience the consequences of engaging in the behavior to learn whether the behavior is likely to result in adverse or desirable outcomes. Instead, people can learn through *vicarious reinforcement*; observing whether the outcome for the other person is positive or negative, and assessing whether this outcome is desirable will determine if someone is likely to model the behavior. Bandura also proposed that people are more likely to model the behavior of someone who is similar to themselves. With regard to self-injury, this could account for peers modeling the behavior of peers seen to be demographically similar (e.g., the same age) or peers who are struggling with the same mental health concerns or life stressors. Individuals are also more likely to model the behavior of people they respect, admire, or aspire to be like. This could explain increases in suicides that can occur after reports of celebrity suicides. Although less work has explored the effect of celebrities disclosing a history of self-injury, it is likely that people who admire these celebrities may be at increased risk of self-injury, as they emulate the behavior of their idols.

In the 1980s Bandura expanded his social learning theory to include a cognitive component. In proposing social cognitive theory,[28] he recognized that one thing that makes humans unique among animals is the ability to forecast the future, and imagine what may happen if they were to engage in a given behavior. As such, even without having ever engaged in a behavior people can formulate an expectation about what the outcome might be. These outcome expectancies are evaluated, such that if a positive outcome is anticipated, one is more likely to engage in a behavior, and if a negative outcome is anticipated they are less likely to engage in the behavior. Similar to vicarious learning, people can learn these outcome expectancies by observing the outcomes that occur when other people engage in a behavior. For example, if a child sees their mother stressed after a busy day at work who then says "I need a drink" and proceeds to pour a glass of wine, the child will develop an outcome expectancy that alcohol reduces stress. In the future, they are then more likely to pour themselves a drink when they feel stressed.

Few studies have explored the development of outcome expectancies related to self-injury. We[29] outlined an explicit role for self-injury outcome expectancies in our cognitive emotional model of self-injury, proposing that people bring these expectancies with them to any given situation. In an emotionally volatile situation, an individual is more likely to self-injure if they expect self-injury will result in favorable outcomes (e.g., reducing distress), and less likely to self-injure if they expect unfavorable outcomes (e.g., physical pain). We later[5] tested this proposition, and observed that holding positive outcome expectancies was related to an increased probability of self-injury, while negative outcome expectancies about self-injury reduced the probability of self-injury. In another study,[30] we tested five specific outcome expectancies related to self-injury: expectations of affect regulation, physical pain, anticipated negative self-beliefs (e.g., I would feel like a failure), anticipated negative social consequence (e.g., My friends would be disgusted), and expectations about communication (e.g., Other people would notice and offer sympathy). Individuals with a history of self-injury held stronger expectations of affect regulation, and weaker expectations that self-injury would be painful, than individuals with no such history.

Although Bandura proposed these outcome expectancies may be learned by observing the outcomes of others engaging in a behavior, only a handful of studies have explored how outcome expectancies might work in concert with observation of self-injury. In other work, we[5] observed that knowing a friend who self-injures, the number of friends who self-injure, and positive outcome expectancies were each related to increased probability of one's own self-injury, but they did not work together to increase this risk. Dawkins and colleagues[31] asked university students to report whether they had a parent with a history of self-injury. Knowing a parent who self-injured conferred a threefold increase in the probability that the student self-injured. However, this relation was mediated by expectations of pain and affect regulation. Specifically, if a parent self-injured the student held stronger affect regulation expectancies, and weaker expectations of pain, which in turn were related to increased probability of self-injury. This might suggest that students have learned these outcome expectancies by observing, or talking about, self-injury with parents, although further work is needed to confirm this hypothesis.

IATROGENIC EFFECTS IN INTERVENTION AND PREVENTION

Iatrogenic effects concern ill health that is the result of medical treatment. In the context of self-injury, there is concern that group treatment may increase risk of self-injury (produce an iatrogenic effect), due to potential socialization effects within therapy groups. Specifically, if individuals in treatment discuss their self-injury in detail, there is potential for people to gain knowledge of new ways to self-injure, to compete with others they believe to be engaging in more severe self-injury, learn new ways to hide their self-injury from others, or to be triggered by their own underlying distress. Likewise, schools express concern that addressing self-injury in prevention initiatives may increase risk of students starting to self-injure.

An early randomized controlled trial of group therapy for self-harm (broadly defined) reported promising results with reductions in the repetition of self-harm.[32] Several other randomized controlled trials of group therapy for self-injury have failed to show effects in the reduction of frequency or repetition of self-injury, but also failed to show increases in the behavior, suggesting a lack of iatrogenic effects.[33,34] These treatments did not focus exclusively on self-injury but addressed related concerns such as relationship and peer problems, anger management, depression, and hopelessness. This broader focus may have precluded detailed discussion of self-injury, and thus reduced risk of iatrogenic effects.

Similarly, emotion regulation group therapy, designed as an adjunct to treatment as usual, focuses on deficits in core areas of emotion regulation (acceptance of emotion, awareness of emotion, clarity of emotion, goal-directed behavior, impulse control, emotion regulation strategies). This program has demonstrated successful reductions of self-injury, particularly in samples of women diagnosed with borderline personality disorder.[35,36] In a small trial ($n = 19$) of voice and movement therapy for self-injury,[37] no changes in self-injury were observed, although there were improvements in emotion regulation, alexithymia, self-esteem, and psychological distress. Throughout the 10-week program, two participants were briefly admitted to psychiatric wards following suicide attempts and one was accompanied to the emergency department with acute distress, dissociation, and suicidal ideation following a session. Clearly, even if the risk is low, clinicians must be mindful of the potential for adverse events related to group treatment and have an adverse events protocol in place.

Cases of social circulation of self-injury have been particularly noted in closed settings such as hospitals.[38] This is most likely to occur in small group interactions, as a display of affinity between two people.[38,39] In a study involving adolescents in an inpatient setting, Zhu and colleagues[12] noted that more frequent exposure to specific methods was related to greater use of that method to self-injure, however it is not clear whether exposure was in the context of the hospital, with many reporting exposure to self-injury before engaging in the behavior themselves. Analysis of data obtained from a 5-year retrospective cohort study on peer influences on self-harm (broadly defined) in an adolescent inpatient unit found that spontaneous occurrence of self-harm was infrequent, and that those with a history of self-harm tended to reduce the frequency of the behavior while in hospital.[40]

With regard to prevention, an open trial of the Signs of Self-Injury prevention program, conducted across five secondary schools, demonstrated increased knowledge, improved help-seeking attitudes and intentions, but no iatrogenic effects among students.[41] The program includes psychoeducation about self-injury, but also maintains a focus on supporting students who self-injure and reducing stigma. Screening programs designed to detect students at elevated risk of self-injury or suicidal behavior also do not appear to elevate distress among students, and appear to be acceptable to students, parents, and staff.[42] Overall, if conducted well, primary prevention programs do not appear to confer iatrogenic effects.

IATROGENIC EFFECTS IN RESEARCH

There has been a growing body of work exploring the potential for iatrogenic effects to occur as a result of participating in research about self-injury and suicidal thoughts and behaviors. Specifically, there has been some concern that by answering questions about self-injury in surveys or interviews, or reflecting on self-injury reported by friends, that vulnerable people might be more susceptible to self-injury—that reflection on these research questions gives people the idea to self-injure. There is additional concern that focus on self-injury, particularly for people with a history of self-injury, may be distressing and increase urges to self-injure. For this reason, ethics committees are often reluctant to approve research focused on self-injury, particularly when the target population of interest is young people. While it is true that young people are more susceptible to peer influence,[43] and potentially at greater risk of self-injury, this work consistently finds that although some people can experience discomfort in answering sensitive questions, the benefits far outweigh the potential risks.

Randomized controlled trials show that rather than produce iatrogenic effects, inclusion of items about self-injury or suicidal thoughts and behaviors actually increases psychological well-being of at risk youth (with a prior history of depression) *more* than youth with no prior history, and more than those who were not administered these items.[44,45] In experimental work, where participants were asked to view repeated presentations of self-injury-related images (e.g., of cut skin) and words (e.g., suicide), a slight decline in mood was noted from some participants but there was no change in urges to self-injure.[46] Instead, people report enjoying participating in research, and report altruistic reasons for doing so (i.e., to help the researchers, help young people[47]). In similar lines of research, participants report that study participation gives them greater insight into themselves.[48] In many studies, young people report significant benefits from research participation.[45,47,49] Participation in research studies may also facilitate support seeking if researchers provide informational and clinical resources to participants; indeed this may be one way to ensure people who self-injure know help is available to them.[47]

Despite a lack of evidence for iatrogenic effects occurring through research participation, researchers do need to be mindful of their duty of care to participants. Numerous guidelines for conducting research about self-injury are available.[50,51] These suggest that to prevent iatrogenic effects researchers can:

1. Use skip logic in online questionnaires, so people are not exposed to self-injury items that are not relevant to them
2. Provide opportunities to take a break when needed
3. In online questionnaires, provide a distraction page (e.g., of unrelated puzzles) that participants can visit when they need a break
4. End the study with a mood induction or relaxation exercise to ensure participants are not experiencing elevated distress as a result of the study
5. Provide general mental health and self-injury-specific resources to all participants

A PERSON-CENTERED APPROACH TO MINIMIZING SOCIALIZATION OF SELF-INJURY

A person-centered approach to addressing and minimizing socialization effects (Table 6.1) requires the acknowledgment that people engage in self-injury for a number of different reasons. Individuals who report social reasons for engaging in self-injury also report emotion regulatory reasons, and social reasons are recognized as the least effective reasons to self-injure. Further, discussion of self-injury among peer groups may serve an important support function, and not automatically increase risk of further self-injury. As such, we recommend avoiding making assumptions about why people self-injure, or assuming that socialization effects naturally follow when peers self-injure.

However, to minimize socialization effects, consideration of who might be at elevated risk of peer influence is important. There is very little research on who is most at risk, but younger adolescents appear to be most susceptible to peer influence, and this tends to coincide with the average age of self-injury onset. Rather than completely avoid discussion of self-injury, we suggest that self-injury is part of a broader conversation about how people cope. Consistent with media guidelines, we recommend limiting explicit discussion of self-injury methods, and

Table 6.1. PRACTICAL TIPS FOR MINIMIZING SOCIALIZATION EFFECTS.

Avoid	Instead
• Detailed discussion of self-injury methods	• Discuss self-injury within a broader context of coping
• Images (stylized or not) of self-injury	• Use images that promote recovery and resilience (e.g., flowers growing out of a desert)
• Group treatment for self-injury	• Engage individuals in a one-on-one treatment, unless the focus is on specific skills building
• Sensationalizing self-injury in media or social media contexts	• Tell stories of recovery that can foster hope and optimism for people who self-injure
• Assuming someone is self-injuring solely to fit in with peers	• Talk with the person about what function self-injury serves for them
• Focusing only on self-injury among peer groups	• Situate discussion of self-injury within a broader social context, including societal attitudes, stigma, and impacts on both the individual and loved ones

avoiding graphic self-injury images. In school settings, students who are engaging in detailed talk of self-injury could be reminded that this might be upsetting or triggering for any peers who are coping with their own concerns. Given the importance of peer relationships for adolescents, this is likely to encourage the young person to seek alternate outlets to express their feelings about self-injury.

Many clinicians have recommended that treatment for self-injury be conducted one-on-one rather than in group settings.[52,53] While we know of cases where an individual has increased their self-injury as a result of group discussion, there are also many cases where there have been no iatrogenic effects of group therapy. Further, given that many individuals who self-injure feel isolated and alienated, group therapies may offer social support and opportunities to model alternative coping strategies. If group therapy is delivered, we again suggest that clinicians refrain from encouraging discussion of self-injury methods or focusing exclusively on self-injury, but instead focus on peer and family relationships, coping strategies, and skills building.[53]

RETHINKING CONTAGION: SOCIAL CAUSES AND SOCIAL CONSEQUENCES OF SELF-INJURY

Throughout this chapter, we have focused on the associations between exposure to self-injury among peers, media, and in clinical or research settings to an individual's own self-injury. However, we suggest that the consideration of the social aspects of self-injury be much broader in scope and cover a range of social causes and consequences of self-injury. Borrowing from the broader field of social psychology, this might include societal attitudes toward self-injury, media coverage of self-injury, stigma toward and attributions about self-injury and individuals who engage in the behavior, the roles of conformity and obedience in selection and socialization effects, identity formation, and cognitive dissonance—particularly in relation to ambivalence that may be experienced when considering reducing or stopping self-injury. Social consequences of self-injury could include: the impact on families, peers, healthcare workers, and school staff; interactions with healthcare staff; help or support seeking; and impacts of any visible scarring on employment, relationships, or a person's activities. We touch on some if these issues in later chapters of this book.

Within this broader framework, there are many more avenues of exploration than simply selection and socialization effects. Together, these lines of inquiry would allow a much more compressive picture of the role of social factors in self-injury, and remove the focus from the problematic notion of "contagion." At its core, this broader framework recognizes that self-injury is not an issue concerned only with the individual, but that it is a societal concern, with many social factors implicated, and affected by, self-injury.

Along similar lines, we recognize that self-injury has a socially constructed meaning. By definition, self-injury is a behavior that is not socially or culturally sanctioned. In defining it this way, it has automatically been given a social meaning—as a behavior that is not accepted, socially divergent, and that may vary in meaning across cultures and time. A shared understanding of self-injury comes from the way society communicates about the behavior including through media and social media, and we must be mindful that this communication does not create a shared understanding that promotes stigma, or shame, among individuals who self-injure. A lens of social constructionism might also help individuals who self-injure ascribe meaning to the behavior, and help work toward an understanding that fosters resilience and self-acceptance.

CONCLUSION

The notion that people can gain the idea to self-injure from peers, media, or social media has prompted anxiety about how best to address self-injury online, in schools, and in clinical settings. While it is true that some people gain the idea to self-injure from others, social bonding does not appear to be a factor in the maintenance of the behavior. Rather than always resulting in socialization effects, discussion of self-injury, in peer groups and online, may foster a sense of belonging and offer opportunities to model alternate coping strategies. As such, there is a fine line to walk in minimizing socialization effects while acknowledging the benefits of sharing experiences of self-injury. We propose that one way to minimize the focus on socialization effects is to broaden the conversation to include the wide range of social causes and social consequences of self-injury.

Self-Injury, the Internet, and Social Media

With the advent of social media, online communication has become central to how people across the globe connect with one another and obtain information. Indeed, people routinely use the Internet to express their identities, share material (e.g., images, video), obtain information and news, affiliate with various causes and social movements, as well as create and maintain social ties.[1-3] Similarly, online communication has become exceedingly relevant to many individuals who self-injure.[4] Although this is the case, several reviews of the literature indicate that online communication about self-injury can yield both potential benefits and risks.[4-6] Thus, the scope and nature of online activity regarding self-injury have come to represent areas of increasing interest and, at times, concern among researchers and mental health professionals.[7-11] In this way, it is important to bear both in mind and to avoid sweeping generalizations that online activity regarding self-injury is *all* good or bad. Rather, a more nuanced and balanced understanding of this literature is needed—one that contextualizes and articulates the reasons people who engage in self-injury use the Internet alongside understanding the potential benefits and risks that may stem from such online activity. The current chapter thus summarizes this growing literature and concludes by offering recommendations about how to use a person-centered approach to engage in conversations about online self-injury activity with people who have lived experience.

REASONS FOR ONLINE SELF-INJURY ACTIVITY

A recent synthesis of the existing literature in this area indicates three principal reasons for online self-injury activity: (1) obtainment of acceptance and validation, (2) curiosity and fostering understanding, and (3) help and support.[12] For the most part, this literature involves instances in which individuals with lived experience of self-injury activity seek out material related to self-injury or to connect with people who similarly self-injure. At the same time, it should not be assumed this is always the case; there are also instances in which people inadvertently access self-injury content (e.g., when browsing major social networks),[7,13,14] which we address later.

Obtainment of Acceptance and Validation

As presented in Chapter 4, people who self-injure commonly report stigmatizing experiences, including negative reactions from others.[15] Because of this, Internet use may afford an ostensibly safe means to connect with others; coupled with this, there may be appeal, and perhaps solace, inherent in finding and communicating with like-minded others—namely, people who also have lived self-injury experience.[16] Hence, these interactions may normalize that one is not alone in the experience of self-injury, which may contribute to a sense of acceptance and validation.[17,18]

Reports of individuals receiving acceptance and validation for their self-injury experiences have been documented in several studies. For example, a recent investigation of self-injury content on Instagram found that people may upload self-injury imagery with the aim of being validated by other community members,[19] similar to what has been reported across other platforms such as YouTube and self-injury discussion fora.[9,20,21] In these cases, part of the Internet's appeal is likely attributable to the (seemingly) anonymous nature of communication it affords.[8,9,14,16,22] Indeed, researchers have found that people with lived self-injury experience report more difficulty speaking about self-injury with people in their offline lives (e.g., family) than when talking to people (often who they do not know) online.[17] This may be due to prior experiences in which self-injury was poorly responded to, a sense that people in one's life will not understand self-injury, or perhaps a view that the nature of online interactions are simpler, given their absence of complexities more typical of existing relationships (e.g., concerns about changing the quality of the relationship, worry about losing a relationship altogether).

Curiosity and Fostering Understanding

Much like the Internet is used to find information for various health-related topics, researchers have found that individuals who engage in self-injury go online to obtain information and learn about self-injury.[13,14,23,24] Indeed, searches for self-injury via the Internet occur at very high volumes and occur widely geographically. For example, one of our studies estimated that searches for self-injury content on Google occur well over 40 million times annually.[24] Given the increased attention on self-injury since that study was published in 2014, it is reasonable to surmise this number is higher today.

In some cases, seeking information may factor into people's reasons for online self-injury activity. For example, in another one of our studies asking people with lived experience of self-injury about reasons for their online activity, participants reported that a common reason for initially going online was to learn more about self-injury in order to develop a deeper understanding of their own experience.[14] Commensurate with this, other researchers have found that people who self-injure may go online to seek information about self-injury before taking part in other forms of online activities, such as communication with others.[13] Seeking information about self-injury is thus salient for many individuals, perhaps even contributing to the initiation of online self-injury activity.

Receiving and Provision of Support

People who engage in self-injury may also go online to get support.[14,16,21–24,26] In the majority of cases, the nature of support sought tends to be more informal in nature; that is, individuals do not necessarily go online with an explicit desire to necessarily stop self-injuring or obtain professional help; rather, they seek non-judgmental support (e.g., encouragement that one can recover) and validation (e.g., acknowledgement that they are not alone in their experience) from others. Accordingly, the support sought is from other individuals who have lived experience of self-injury.[14,16,23,26] There are likely several reasons for this. As noted previously, stigma may drive people to seek acceptance and connection with others with whom they can relate. In some cases, this may stem from previous disheartening experiences and interactions with others. It may also be that individuals believe that only people who have self-injured can fully understand and offer support to other individuals who have self-injured.[23]

In addition, individuals who self-injure may use the Internet to *offer* support to others. During their interactions with others, people who self-injure may develop a sense of solidarity and may even form online friendships. When this occurs, it may contribute to a willingness to engage in reciprocal support, with some people specifically going online for this purpose.[21,22] Thus, while more research is needed in this area, the obtainment *and* provision of support represent key reasons for online self-injury activity.

Other Reasons for Online Self-Injury Activity

Although the reasons discussed above are the most cited in the literature, others warrant mentioning. As reported in a recent summary of the field,[12] these include, but are not necessarily limited to: the opportunity to freely articulate one's experiences without interruption or filtering; the practical and accessible means of online communication (e.g., people can go online on their own time); and advocacy-related purposes such as debunking common misconceptions linked to self-injury (e.g., the common misperception that only girls self-injure).[16,21,22] Other research points to the importance of people documenting their experiences with self-injury. In particular, some studies have found that individuals go online to share aspects of their self-injury experiences, including setbacks (e.g., recurrences of self-injury), urges to self-injure, and progress in recovery (e.g., discussing how one did not act on an urge or noting the time from the last time they self-injured).[21,22,27] It should therefore be evident that while there are commonly reported reasons for engagement in online self-injury activity, it cannot be assumed that any one reason necessarily applies to any one person. Much like we noted in Chapter 1 when discussing reasons for self-injury engagement, one's reasons for online communication about self-injury may likewise change over time.

PERCEIVED BENEFITS OF INTERNET USE FOR INDIVIDUALS WHO SELF-INJURE

Now that we have established what may motivate people with lived experience of self-injury to engage in online activity related to self-injury, we turn to a discussion of the possible benefits this may have. Several comprehensive reviews[4-6] have reported on the ways that online self-injury activity may impact those involved. Based on this collection of evidence as well as studies published following these reviews, four primary benefits of online self-injury activity have been documented, namely: (1) mitigation of social isolation; (2) disclosure; (3) reductions in self-injury; (4) recovery encouragement and resource provision.[12]

Mitigation of Social Isolation

The most commonly reported benefit of online self-injury activity throughout the academic literature is that, when online, individuals with lived self-injury experience feel less socially isolated.[4,27,28] As discussed earlier, many people who self-injure experience stigma and are often the recipients of unhelpful (at times, hurtful) responses from others.[15] which can, in turn, foment loneliness, shame, and isolation.[15,29,30] By virtue of going online and reading about others' experience or interacting with other people, individuals who self-injure may begin to feel more supported;[4,20,23,31] in short, underlying needs for acceptance, validation, and emotional support may be at least partially met when online.[4,12] Of note, people with lived experience may find utility in connecting with others who also self-injure. In support of this are research findings indicating that some individuals who self-injure prefer connecting with others who also self-injure.[14] In this way, receiving compassionate, nonjudgmental responses from like-minded others may be invaluable. Interacting with online peers may therefore offer a sense of connection and community,[23,24,32–34] which lessens feelings of aloneness.[16,23,24] In summary, isolation and feelings of aloneness may be thwarted through a number of mechanisms,[12] including but not limited to supportive understanding (i.e., obtaining support from people with similar experiences), relational bonds (i.e., fostering connections with others), and reciprocal support (i.e., provision and obtainment of positive feedback, interaction, and support).[12,23]

Disclosure

As a result of their inbuilt anonymity (or potential for this), many online platforms arguably represent appealing contexts in which to share otherwise difficult experiences. Findings from a number of studies support this in the context of self-injury, with people who self-injure indicating that they feel more comfortable and willing to share their self-injury experiences and associated feelings via the Internet than in offline settings.[10,35–37] There may also be a communal aspect tied to disclosing one's experience; that is, disclosing one's experiences online may invite others to do the same. For instance, in a follow-up study to one of our studies investigating the content of self-injury videos on YouTube,[9] we found that the most common type of comment to self-injury videos involved sharing one's own experiences with self-injury.[20] It is possible that this kind of experience-sharing reflects the need to unmask parts of the self and one's self-injury.[4] Indeed, the Internet may be a means by which to share one's authentic self with others.[32] In sum, people who have self-injured may benefit from the Internet in that it permits the sharing of otherwise concealed aspects of their experience and identities.

Reductions in Self-Injury

Although a dearth of research has explored the link between online activity and self-injury engagement, some researchers have indicated that involvement in certain forms of online activities may associate with less frequent self-injury and improvements in coping with difficult psychological experiences. [16,24,33] For example, in one study, over half of participants indicated less frequent self-injury engagement pursuant to joining an online community.[33] There are likely a few reasons to account for these reports. Part of this may stem from the opportunity these fora provide in terms of operating as an emotional outlet and vehicle of expression,[23] which may work to curb self-injury enactment.[33] It is also possible that use of the Internet allows individuals to distract themselves from self-injury urges, thereby allowing for self-injury urges to diminish in intensity; if this is the case, it would cohere with clinical recommendations that outline strategies to help individuals resist acting on self-injury urges.[38] Consistent with this, another possibility is that when online, people are exposed to strategies and suggestions about ways to cope with urges and how to manage self-injury more generally.[4] Although the precise means by which reductions in self-injury can occur by way of online activity is not clear, it seems that the Internet may be associated with decreases in self-injury and improved coping for a subset of individuals. At the same time, as addressed a bit later, certain forms of online activity related to self-injury may also carry risks for continued self-injury.[4]

Recovery Encouragement and Resource Provision

A common topic of self-injury related conversation in online arenas is the aspect of recovery.[4] Although the nature of what is discussed about recovery varies considerably (e.g., discussing it as possible or not), in some cases, individuals may be encouraged to engage in recovery efforts while receiving hopeful messages from others.[4,6] Congruently, several online platforms have been reported to provide self-injury coping strategies as well as promote help and support-seeking offline.[4,6,34,39,40] Thus, online communication between members may encourage recovery through both informal means (e.g., peer support, provision of resources) and more formal means by way of encouraging people to seek help and support in their offline lives. Although scant research has directly examined the benefits of accessing recovery-oriented content online, there is some preliminary support from one of our studies to indicate that exposure to hopeful messages about recovery may contribute to more positive views about one's own recovery prospects.[41]

PERCEIVED RISKS OF ONLINE COMMUNICATION

As documented throughout the literature, and noted earlier, online self-injury activities represent a double-edged sword.[4] Thus, while there are several noted benefits, there are also potential risks. A survey of the existing evidence, comprising comphrensive reviews[4-6] and a recent consolidation of the literature[12] highlights three major risks linked to online self-injury activity: (1) self-injury engagement and reinforcement, (2) triggering of self-injury urges, and (3) stigmatization.

Engagement and Reinforcement of Self-Injury

Of the risks identified in the literature, self-injury engagement and reinforcement is the most frequently cited.[4,12] In short, this involves the potential for certain kinds of online activity related to self-injury associating with engagement in, and specifically repetition of, self-injury. For instance, studies have indicated that on some websites people share tips and strategies about how to hide self-injury from others (e.g., family) or even ways to self-injure that have a low likelihood of being discovered.[8,11] Researchers have similarly found that self-injury first-aid strategies (e.g., preparing for an self-injury episode, cleaning wounds after self-injury) are frequently shared online.[8,42] Access to these kinds of strategies could conceivably contribute to further self-injury and impede help or support-seeking. In support of this, our research examining self-injury content on YouTube has found that only a small fraction of videos overtly mentioned help-seeking.[8,20,42]

In addition, the portrayal of self-injury online has been suggested to glamorize self-injury itself. This may occur when self-injury is linked to high-profile celebrities who may be idolized[8] or when photos of self-injury are uploaded and shared online.[43] With the latter, concerns have been expressed that certain imagery may render self-injury engagement more desirable to vulnerable individuals.[8] For example, graphic photos with emotionally charged captions may accrue numerous views (and comments), which may render self-injury more appealing for certain at-risk individuals; thus, it may provoke others to post their own images. In a similar manner, researchers have reported that these kinds of presentations as well as how self-injury is presented in text-based descriptions online, may normalize the behavior as a justified means to cope with distress.[44] Should these types of messages resonate with people who access them, they may contribute to continued self-injury.[4]

Related to the manner by which self-injury is presented online are reports that self-injury is often situated in the context of hopeless themes, including suggestions that recovery is impossible or pointless. Unfortunately, these messages are common across self-injury websites[8] and on social media.[9,20] In some cases, these messages are also packaged in the context of self-injury being perceived as an addiction; here, people post messages about feeling addicted to self-injury, which renders the prospect of recovery quite difficult.[45] Notwithstanding the contention of viewing self-injury as an addiction[45,46] these kinds of messages are widely accessible online.[11,45]

Collectively, repeated access to the above types of messages has been thought to exacerbate existing feelings of helplessness and hopelessness, and, as a consequence, deter efforts to obtain support or work toward recovery.[4,12,45] Despite the impact this kind of content might have, some research has found that even when individuals who self-injure acknowledge that repeated access to melancholic and hopeless material is upsetting, they nonetheless continue going online.[14] Therefore, not only are hopeless messages about self-injury recovery prevalent, they may be continually accessed despite their potential adverse impact. It has also been suggested that some individuals may be accessing this kind of content as a form of self-punishment, perhaps akin to some people's reasons for self-injury.

Clearly, more research is needed to better understand the reasoning and impact of accessing these kinds of hopeless messages.

The above reports tend to apply to individuals who already engage in self-injury and who actively seek out online material related to self-injury. However, there is some evidence to suggest that exposure to self-injury material online may contribute to self-injury engagement, among individuals who have self-injured and even individuals who have no prior self-injury history. In a prospective study involving young adults who accessed self-injury content on Instagram, viewing self-injury imagery was found to associate with self-injury as well as suicidal ideation and emotion difficulties.[7] This was not only the case at the initial timepoint but also at follow-up—and, at follow-up, this applied to individuals with a prior self-injury history as well as those without. Moreover, this trend was found for individuals who were not even seeking out self-injury material on Instagram (i.e., exposure to self-injury material was accidental). Although causality cannot be assumed, these findings offer some preliminary evidence that certain vulnerable individuals may be at risk for self-injury pursuant to accessing self-injury content online. How and when this transpires remains unclear. It is therefore critical to bear in mind that exposure to self-injury content in itself is insufficient to contribute to self-injury enactment.[46,47] The relation is much more complex and likely involves several factors and psychological processes.

Triggering

Several reports have been made with respect to an individual's online self-injury communication and the potential for this to provoke (trigger) distress, urges to self-injure and, in some cases, self-injury engagement.[4] For example, between 11% and 33% of individuals who maintain self-injury webpages have reported feeling triggered after viewing online content.[8,22] In particular, viewing graphic self-injury images or reading detailed descriptions of others' self-injury experiences have been tied to the potential for triggering effects.[4,12] For these reasons, and across many websites, individuals and site moderators post "trigger warnings" in an effort to flag particular material as potentially upsetting. Perhaps unsurprisingly, there is little evidence these efforts work to dissuade individuals from accessing the flagged material. Moreover, their effectiveness in terms of minimizing distress is not well supported; in other words, seeing a trigger warning prior to viewing material has little to no impact on the level of ensuring distress experienced.[48] The impact that graphic self-injury content may have has been debated among individuals who take part in online self-injury activity, with some people vehemently opposed to imagery and other graphic material being posted at all and others discussing the need to freely express themselves.[43]

Notwithstanding the above reports, not all self-injury content affects people in the same manner—even material that has been linked to triggering effects. For example, in one of our studies examining how individuals with a self-injury history discussed reactions to viewing self-injury photos online, some users reported decreases in self-injury urge intensity subsequent to seeing such imagery.[43] In addition, there may be marked differences in a user's reaction to photos of self-injury-related scars versus injuries, with some people finding injuries, but not scarring, triggering.[43] While these reports warrant replication and inquiry into explanatory mechanisms, these findings imply that individuals may be differentially impacted by online self-injury material.

Stigmatization

Due to the stigma associated with self-injury, the Internet may serve as a much needed refuge for individuals who self-injure.[4] Yet, online self-injury activity may also expose people to stigma through negative comments from others. In support of this, researchers examining self-injury groups on Facebook found that demeaning and critical posts were present in just over 20% of the groups studied.[34] Similar reports have been made in other research examining self-injury content on Facebook.[44] Unfortunately, these kinds of posts are not unique to Facebook. Hostile and otherwise stigmatizing comments toward people who self-injure have been observed in comments to self-injury videos on YouTube[20] and in responses to people's requests for support and validation on *Yahoo!* Answers.[18] In addition to exposure to others' comments, stigmatization may also occur through the presentation of self-injury information, such as material intended to provide facts or information about self-injury. In research examining the quality of websites retrieved through common Google searches for self-injury content, it has been found that a majority of websites were composed of poor-quality information which propagated at least one self-injury myth (e.g., only adolescents self-injure).[25,49] This kind of misinformation can inadvertently communicate that others (who do not self-injure) do not understand self-injury. As people who self-injure are acutely aware of self-injury myths and how the behavior is often perceived,[51] seeing a broader discourse in which self-injury is misrepresented has the potential to exacerbate existing feelings of being misunderstood and marginalized.[25]

A PERSON-CENTERED-BASED CONTEXTUALIZATION

An important part of understanding online self-injury communication is first recognizing the vital role it plays for many people with lived experience.

Considering the significant stigma tied to self-injury,[15] the sense of isolation common to many people's experience, and concerns about the reaction of people in their offline lives, many individuals draw on their inner resources to reach out to others via the Internet.[10,16,21,37] Understanding the functionality of online communication is thus critical. This is not to say that we ignore the complicated nature of online self-injury activity, however. There are indeed both potential benefits *and* risks linked to accessing certain kinds of self-injury content.[4] A balanced approach is therefore needed—one that takes into account the full range of risks *and* benefits associated with online self-injury activity, that avoids assumptions or confirmatory biases (e.g., the common view that all online self-injury activity is harmful), and allows for *open* conversations with individuals with lived self-injury experience.

Although discussions about online self-injury activity vary by context (e.g., parents with teens versus clinicians with clients), in general, acknowledging and validating that online self-injury activity serves a purpose for individuals is vital. Doing so allows for more open dialogue about the topic, which some individuals who self-injure may be initially reluctant to do.[18,28] To facilitate these conversations, adopting a nonjudgmental respectful curiosity[52-54] (see Chapter 2) is advised. This positions individuals who self-injure as the expert in *their* experience (e.g., *can you help me understand what your online activity related to self-injury does for you?*), which can translate to a greater willingness for individual with lived experience to engage in conversation. As these discussions may sometimes occur in clinical settings (i.e., between mental health professionals and clients) we recommend that mental health professionals draw on published guidelines for use when assessing online self-injury activity and incorporating this into clinical work.[12,28]

One issue that often arises in discourses about online self-injury activity is whether online self-injury material ought to be banned. While a full discussion about social media policy is beyond the scope of this book (e.g., news stories about Instagram or Facebook banning self-injury content), suggestions or even efforts to ban people's access to online material related to self-injury are bound to be unhelpful and may work to exacerbate people's feelings of being marginalized and shunned from society. Rather than overtly discouraging online activity, it can be useful to provide a list of potentially helpful online resources which may have appeal to individuals with lived nonsuicidal self-injury (NSSI) experience. With this in mind, Table 7.1 presents websites with recovery-oriented resources (e.g., coping strategies, access to hopeful stories about recovery). For social media platforms, drawing on recently developed media guidelines—that include guidance for social media—is also advised.[55]

Table 7.1. RECOMMENDED RESOURCES FOR PEOPLE WITH LIVED EXPERIENCE OF SELF-INJURY. IN SOME CASES, THESE CAN BE SHARED WITH OTHER STAKEHOLDERS (E.G., WITH FAMILIES WHEN WORKING WITH MINORS).

Website Name & URL	Description
Self-Injury Outreach and Support (SiOS) www.sioutreach.org	SiOS has numerous research-informed resources about self-injury tailored to people who have self-injured, including coping guides and recovery stories from those with lived experience. In addition to this, SiOS offers guides for families, friends, romantic partners, schools, and various health and mental professionals.
Cornell Research Program on Self-Injury and Recovery www.selfinjury.bctr.cornell.edu	Based at Cornell University, this website provides an array of resources concerning self-injury. This includes resources for people who self-injure, including material on recovery. Additionally, this website has information for families, schools, and professionals.
SAFE Alternatives www.selfinjury.com	SAFE Alternatives is a treatment approach and service located in the United States. Their website also houses educational resources for individuals engaging in NSSI, caregivers, families, and educational and health professionals.
Shedding Light on Self-Injury www.self-injury.org.au	This online resource has information for health professionals, as well as general information for anyone wanting more information about self-injury.
The Mighty's Guide to Understanding Self-Harm https://themighty.com/ 2019/06/what-is-self-harm/ #addiction-self-harm	This webpage is part of The Mighty, an online community with the aim of connecting and empowering people with lived experience of physical and mental health difficulties. This page of the website offers consolidated information about self-injury for individuals with lived experience of self-injury (youth and young adult) as well as material for concerned loved ones.

NOTE: This table mirrors Box 13.2 as the websites listed are relevant to readers of both chapters.

CONCLUSION

As can be seen in this chapter, the use of the Internet by individuals with lived self-injury experience has emerged as a major area of research and one that has numerous implications.[4–6] There are many reasons that drive this kind of online activity and there are many ways that people may be impacted—both positively and negatively—by online self-injury activity. Indeed, it is not as straightforward as blanketing online self-injury activity as "harmful" or "helpful." However, by using a person-centered approach that avoids generalizations and appreciates the nuances of online activity related to self-injury, we will be better positioned to not just understand this complex literature but also engage in more effective conversations with, and ultimately support, people who have lived experience of self-injury.

Addressing Self-Injury in Schools

A Student-Centered, Strengths-Based Approach

ROLES PEOPLE PLAY IN SCHOOLS

In school settings, self-injury is associated with symptoms of depression and anxiety, poor peer relationships, and deteriorating academic performance.[1,2] However, supportive school environments offer a protective effect, reducing the chance of self-injury.[3,4] Successfully addressing and responding to self-injury in schools requires a whole-of-school approach. This means that every single person working and studying at the school has a dedicated role to play.

School Administrators

One of the most powerful roles belongs to the education departments, school boards, and school principals. It is the administrative level of a school system that sets the priorities for education, including the import given to social and emotional well-being. An administrative system that recognizes that mental health of students is critical to academic performance will embrace mental health promotion and foster well-being among students. Administrators then have the opportunity to adopt a strengths-based approach at a departmental level. This top-down message sets a tone for all schools, subsequently making student-focused mental health a priority for all who work in schools. Concretely, policies and procedures developed at a governmental or school board level have potential to exert the greatest impact, especially if effectively implemented in all schools covered by that jurisdiction. We outline key features of appropriate self-injury protocol later in this chapter.

Unfortunately, school administrators appear divided on the role they play in the social emotional well-being of their students. In a recent study, we interviewed 30 school principals in Australia and Canada regarding their views on the role principals play in addressing and responding to self-injury in schools.[5] Approximately half the principals adopted an academic lens for their school community, with the other half prioritizing social and emotional well-being. The principals with a social emotional lens were more knowledgeable about self-injury, understood the association between mental health and academic performance, and talked about fostering all areas of child development. In contrast, principals adopting an academic lens were focused on standardized test results, lack of resources (financial and staffing), and other behavioral concerns that were viewed as "more important" than self-injury. Regardless of the pedagogical stance, almost all principals delegated to the school's mental health professional (if they had one) when it came to how best to respond to a student who self-injured.

Mental Health Professionals

Mental health staff have a number of different roles to play in schools. These include but are not necessarily limited to: arranging psychoeducation for students, staff, and parents; advocating for self-injury being positioned as a priority in schools; offering individualized treatment for students who self-injure; working with caregivers of youth who self-injure; and/or liaising with external youth agencies.[6-8] Yet, it is surprising that only 1 in 5 mental health professionals have received any education about self-injury.[9] In early work, school counselors were noted as the go-to people for consultation about self-injury,[10] but fewer than 50% felt appropriately qualified to address self-injury.[11] While knowledge about self-injury has significantly improved, mental health professionals are still calling for greater training.[12] However, although often lacking confidence, the majority of school mental health staff do an excellent job of supporting students who self-injure, and parents report feeling supported by school counselors.[13]

Teachers, Coaches, and Others Who Interact With Students

A different role is held by teachers, coaches, and others who interact with students on a daily basis. While not expected to take on the role of a mental health professional, these staff arguably have the most contact with students, and are thus best placed to notice changes in a student's demeanor, strained peer relations, fluctuations in concentration, changes in academic performance, and signs of self-injury (including inappropriate clothing for the season, reluctance to engage in sports that expose skin, and wounds or scars). These staff also have the opportunity to notice signs of strength among students, and can reward positive changes and growth (e.g., increased interaction with peers, engagement in the classroom). Adolescents identify teachers as a source of support, suggesting that if a peer notices or hears that someone has self-injured they could inform a teacher.[14] Despite this, teachers do not feel they have the necessary skills to respond to a student who self-injures. Given principals' deference to mental health professionals when it comes to student well-being, teachers and coaches are the staff least likely to be offered training and professional development opportunities. Strained resources within schools contribute to this lack of training, although provision of support to replace teachers with substitute staff for the duration of the training could help.

In one of our early studies, almost 70% of teachers said they had encountered at least one student who had self-injured; 80% said they had never received any education related to self-injury. Although one-third of teachers immediately refer to a mental health professional, approximately one-third will conduct a risk assessment and provide counseling.[15] Teachers confirm to us that they feel underequipped to work with students who self-injure and 80% would like opportunities to receive more education and training.[15-17] Reaching out to offer training to teachers could be a significant step forward in fostering an appropriate response to self-injury in schools.

Parents and Guardians

Parental support is one of the most salient factors in recovery from self-injury.[18,19] For this reason, where possible, primary caregivers should be involved in decisions regarding the care of students who self-injure. However, school staff must be mindful that a disrupted or unsafe home environment may also be a contributing factor in the reasons a young person is self-injuring, and involving caregivers could inadvertently increase risk for the student. Further, students may experience this break in confidentiality as undermining trust, and further increase any distress they have about their self-injury being discovered.[20] It is imperative that the student is informed when a caregiver is notified of their self-injury, and actively involved in this process. This will empower the student and may open communication pathways between the school, the student, and the caregiver.

While family environments can impact youth who self-injure, self-injury can also impact caregivers and the broader family.[21] Many caregivers are unaware their child is self-injuring and it is not uncommon for them to react with shock, fear, and guilt, as well as concern for their child. Prior to learning of their child's self-injury parents report good family functioning, a view at odds with that reported by youth.[13] Parents of youth who self-injure report significantly greater caregiver strain (e.g., disrupted routines, feeling resentful, feeling guilty) than parents of youth with no mental health concerns.[22] Schools can play a role in supporting parents, including by providing psychoeducation regarding the reasons their child may be self-injuring, appropriate parenting responses (i.e., not overmonitoring or minimizing the behavior), and fostering realistic expectations about recovery.[23] While some school staff maintain their primary concern is the welfare of the student, not their caregivers, parents have told us they would appreciate more support from schools for their own well-being.[24]

Youth Who Self-Injure, and Their Peers

Perhaps the most important people within a school environment are the students—both those who self-injure and their peers. Relationships with peers are particularly influential during adolescence. In longitudinal work, young people who report peer victimization and poor social self-worth are at increased odds of later engaging in self-injury.[25] Similarly, daily hassles with peers are related to frequency of self-injury.[26] Conversely, social support from peers appears to be protective.[19]

Thus, students have a role to play in supporting each other, either in formal peer mentoring roles or in friendship groups. Many students recognize the role they can play in supporting those who self-injure, suggesting students can talk and listen to each other, facilitate communication with trusted adults, increase awareness of self-injury, and help reduce stigma associated with self-injury.[14] Students we spoke to also recognize an advantage in seeking support from friends within the school environment, rather than online, as online communication was thought to be open to misinterpretation. Yet, this support role can be complex, with students reporting that being in a support role can result in significant distress and sense of responsibility.[27] It is incumbent on schools to not just support students who self-injure but also make support available to peers who care about them.

STAFF TRAINING

Given staff are asking for more training related to self-injury, we must ask the question: What does this training look like? In our work, school staff say they would like to see training programs include practical strategies for talking with students who self-injure, clarification of the roles of different personnel in the school, appropriate referral processes, and psychoeducation that dispels myths about self-injury;[9] you'll note that we recommend all these as core elements of any self-injury protocol (see Table 8.1).

Unfortunately, there is very little scientific evaluation of what works when training staff to appropriately address and respond to self-injury in schools. A growing body of work confirms mental health literacy improves confidence in assisting someone with a mental illness, increases help provided to others, and facilitates help-seeking behavior.[28] Gatekeeper training programs are popular in suicide prevention. In these programs, teachers are trained to be on the lookout for warning signs of suicidal thinking, and learn to appropriately refer suicidal students. These are effective in increasing knowledge about suicide, and increasing confidence in responding to students who may be suicidal.[29,30] However, it is important to make a clear distinction between self-injury and suicidal thoughts and behaviors (see Chapter 2). Promising work from Germany suggests that provision of a 2-day workshop to school teachers, and school mental health staff, can improve self-injury-related knowledge, and perceived confidence in skills to respond

Table 8.1. KEY ELEMENTS OF A SCHOOL POLICY.

Clear delineation of roles	The roles of all school staff in responding to self-injury can be outlined so staff are clear in their responsibilities. Ideally a point person (or team) will be appointed as the primary contact point; this person should be capable of case management as well as school-wide education and training.
Risk assessment	Given links between NSSI and suicidal thoughts and behaviors, the point person should be capable of assessing suicide risk. Suicidal thoughts fluctuate over time, so capacity to conduct ongoing assessments is important.
Strengths assessment	Following a strengths-based approach the point person should include an assessment of strengths the student has that can be harnessed in fostering positive change.
Appropriate referral	The point person should be familiar with external services and the appropriate referral pathways for young people who self-injure. Any referral should be done with the involvement of both the student and, where possible, their family.
Involvement of families	For some school staff there may be a tension between maintaining confidentiality of the student and the need to notify their primary caregivers of the behavior. Where possible and safe to do so, families should be involved in decisions affecting both the care, and the education, of their child. It is even more important to include the child in decisions that affect them, ensuring they feel empowered and have agency in their own care plan. This involvement of the student can build further resilience, and applaud the role of the student in their recovery process.
Consideration of social causes and consequences of self-injury	Given that some students gain the idea to self-injure from peers, schools need to be mindful of how self-injury is discussed in group settings. Self-injury should never be discussed in explicit details, and images of NSSI should be avoided. Instead of focusing on self-injury we suggest schools talk about a range of coping strategies students might use, and the need to be empathic and respectful of the choices students make in this regard.

to students who self-injure.[31] These gains were maintained at 6-month follow-up, at which point participants also reported changes in their own behavior.

Much more work is required to determine the best format in which to deliver staff training. A critical component of successful implementation of school-based training is consideration of the needs, and available resources of the school. In our work, although school staff are crying out for additional information and training, they are also calling for additional staff and resources to help address mental health concerns in schools.[9] Mirroring the idea that a whole-of-school approach is the most effective way to address self-injury in schools, school staff tell us that families, and the students themselves, should be involved in any education and training. School nurses have also stressed that a successful approach to addressing self-injury in schools requires a supportive community, including support from the principal.[32] School staff suggest workshops that focus on psychoeducation and referral, delivered yearly, would be welcomed.[9] In addition to training in identifying risk factors, or appropriate responding to self-injury, such training could emphasize the importance of a student-focused approach, recognizing not just factors underpinning self-injury, but also strengths that can be fostered in the school environment.

BOARDING SCHOOLS AND SCHOOL CAMPS

Special mention should be made of how self-injury is addressed in the context of boarding schools, school camps, and other environments where students might be sharing living spaces, be under the care of adults other than their primary caregivers, or have extensive amounts of time in the school environment. There is not much research on self-injury in such environments, but they all contain elements of transition, disruption to usual routine, and distance from family supports, all of which may be distressing and elevate risk of self-injury.[33] Close sleeping and showering arrangements, and group activities such as swimming, may make existing wounds and scars more visible to other students, increasing risk of discovery of a student's self-injury by others. Students can be advised that displaying open wounds may be triggering for other students, but a decision not to conceal scars should be respected[34-36] (see Chapter 11). While discovery or disclosure of self-injury could provide an opportunity to open a dialogue with the student, it may also open the student up to bullying, judgment, and stigma from other students (and staff). School staff can work with students to navigate these difficult situations, and would benefit from self-injury-specific training, whether their primary role is in mental health provision or not.

TALKING SAFELY ABOUT SELF-INJURY IN SCHOOLS

One of the key concerns expressed by schools is the risk that self-injury will "spread" among peer groups, or from student to student. This fear of "social contagion" often prevents schools from discussing self-injury with students, and fosters a culture of fear and shame for students who self-injure.[37] As discussed in Chapter 6, while it is true that some students gain the idea to self-injure from other students, online, or from popular media,[38-40] exposure to self-injury is not sufficient to increase risk of self-injury.[41–43] Still, schools do need to be mindful of the way in which self-injury is discussed. Any content that sensationalizes self-injury, presents images of wounds, glorifies the behavior (e.g., mentioning celebrities who self-injure), or provides detailed discussion of self-injury methods can be triggering for some students and should be avoided. Instead, schools can frame discussion of self-injury within the broader context of coping and well-being, highlighting that there are many different ways students cope with stress.[6] This has the added value of destigmatizing self-injury and facilitating help-seeking.

SCHOOL POLICIES AND PROTOCOLS

With all the different roles present among school staff, students, and parents, effective response to self-injury in schools necessitates a clear policy for how self-injury is addressed. This should be supplemented with a procedural protocol that outlines the appropriate steps to take when a student is known to self-injure. While many schools have policies and protocols in place for addressing suicidal behavior, few have dedicated policy documents for working with students who self-injure. Given the important differences between these behaviors (see Chapter 2), we believe it is critical that a dedicated policy and protocol, separate from any suicide protocol, is developed and made available to all school personnel.

Development of a school self-injury policy provides a means of communicating that the school takes self-injury seriously, as a behavior in its own right, and outlines the ethos of the school when it comes to addressing and responding to self-injury. A good policy document will provide some basic psychoeducation about self-injury and the reasons students might engage in the behavior, and can position a person-centered approach as the guiding framework to addressing self-injury in schools. In such a way, the policy is not simply about the school meeting minimum legal requirements, and not simply duty of care for the students, but becomes a means of advocating a strengths-based approach, upskilling staff, changing attitudes toward self-injury and the students who self-injure, and minimizing stigma in the school setting.

When it comes to procedural steps for working with students who self-injure a clear protocol is required. There are a number of key elements to an effective school protocol.[6,44] These include a recognition that all staff and students have a role to play and clearly delineating the roles that each stakeholder plays; appointment of someone who is able to conduct a suicide risk assessment; in line with a strengths-based approach, an assessment of the strengths, coping resources, and supports a student has at their disposal; a plan for appropriate referral, both within the school and to external service providers if required; consideration of how and when to involve families and caregivers; and consideration of the social causes and consequences of self-injury, including minimizing risk among vulnerable students.

CONCLUSION

Schools offer a unique environment in which to address and respond to self-injury in a way that reduces stigma and promotes empowerment among students. Adopting a whole-of-school approach, in which everyone has a clear role to play, is the most appropriate way to ensure everyone in the school views self-injury as a priority within the school environment, and promotes the same message regarding inclusion and support. Fostering supportive schools, who adopt a strengths-based approach to addressing and responding to self-injury, will go a long way to reducing risk of self-injury and reducing negative consequences for students who do self-injure.

Families and Self-Injury

FAMILIES AS SUPPORTIVE ENVIRONMENTS

Supportive family relationships can serve a protective factor, reducing risk or severity of self-injury. Of note, positive parenting behaviors (e.g., giving praise) are protective against the onset of self-injury,[1] and perceived family support is associated with cessation of self-injury among adolescents.[2] In a daily diary study, university students with more family contact were less likely to self-injure than students with less family contact.[3] Among transgender youth, connectedness with parents can differentiate between youth with a history of self-injury and those without, as well as between youth reporting a suicide attempt and those who did not.[4] Among adolescents, connection with one's parents has been identified as a stronger protective factor than connection with friends.[5] Specifically, adolescents who disclose their self-injury to family report subsequent increases in help-seeking, improved coping, and fewer suicidal thoughts than adolescents who do not talk to their families about self-injury.[6,7]

FAMILIES AS RISK ENVIRONMENTS

Given self-injury is often used to help cope with stress, stressful family environments might pose a risk for self-injury. Argumentative or hostile environments can elevate feelings of self-criticism, rejection, and low self-worth, all of which are risk factors for self-injury. Parental criticism is also associated with self-injury, and over-critical parents may foster self-criticism among individuals who self-injure.[8] In general, poor family support is associated with both the onset and maintenance of self-injury.[9-11] Poor family functioning is associated with heightened emotional reactivity and difficulties regulating emotion, which in turn are associated with self-injury.[12] In fact, poor family functioning can increase risk even for youth who report no difficulties regulating emotion.[13] However, parent and child reports of family functioning differ depending on whether the parent knows about their child engaging in self-injury.[14,15] Young people may also gain the idea to self-injure from siblings who self-injure. As noted in Chapter 6, children of parents who self-injure are three times more likely to self-injure than children who are not aware of a parent's self-injury.[12]

Early childhood trauma, child abuse, parent history of mental health concerns, and poor attachment have all been related to a history of self-injury among adolescents and young adults.[16,17] Physical, sexual, and emotional abuse, as well as neglect, are associated with self-injury.[16] However, the effects appear to be mediated by associated depression and self-blame rather than the maltreatment per se.[18] Likewise, a parental history of mental illness concerns may confer a genetic risk of mental illness among children, which may increase use of self-injury to cope with the psychological symptoms.

WHY DOES ATTACHMENT MATTER?

There are a number of theories regarding how poor attachment can increase risk for self-injury. Linehan[19] maintains that caregivers who do not validate their child's emotions reinforce the notion that emotions are unacceptable. As a result, the child does not learn how to effectively understand and regulate their emotions. Coupled with a high level of impulsivity, this invalidating environment and poor emotion regulation are proposed to be the foundation of borderline personality disorder.[20] As self-injury is one diagnostic feature of borderline personality disorder, this also increases risk of self-injury.

Shore[21] argues that attachment experiences have a direct impact on the formation and development of areas of the brain known to control emotion. These areas are anatomically complete by 15 months of age, but continue to mature through the first two years of life. Furthermore, attachment relationships are associated with later identity formation, which, in turn, is related to self-injury.[22] As such, early bonding experiences with key attachment figures (e.g., parents and caregivers) are critical to later development of effective emotion regulation.

Consistent with this, Fonagy[23] proposed that the understanding of the self is tied to understanding the actions of others. Through observing caregivers and siblings, a child develops an understanding of their own mental states, which Fonagy refers to as *reflective-self functioning* or *mentalization*. Thus, the quality of the attachment relationship is thought to have a direct impact on the child's social and emotional adaptation.[24] Given the affect regulatory role of self-injury, this can then increase risk of self-injury as a means to regulate emotion. Supporting this, individuals who self-injure, report more difficulties with mentalization than people who do not self-injure.[25] In one of the few studies in this area focused specifically on self-injury, recent episodes of self-injury were associated with poorer reflective functioning among adults, but not adolescents.[26]

Fonagy also acknowledges that the caregiver's capacity for mentalization has an impact on the nature of the attachment relationship, and the subsequent emotion regulatory ability of the child. A caregiver who has limited capacity to reflect on their own mental states is more likely to be dismissive or misunderstanding of their child's emotional states, thus creating a poor attachment relationship, and minimizing the opportunities for the child to learn about, understand, and regulate their own emotions. This effect appears particularly pronounced for mothers who have their own trauma experience. Mothers with unresolved trauma exhibit dampened neurological responses to their child's emotions, which may reflect a distancing, or invalidation, of the child's emotional responding.[27]

ATTACHMENT-BASED FAMILY THERAPIES

Due to the role of attachment and family relationships in the onset, maintenance, and cessation of self-injury, there have been calls to trial family therapy in the treatment of self-injury. One potentially relevant approach is attachment-based family therapy, which aims to improve interpersonal relationships by working on the assumption that healing these relationships will lead to a reduction in symptomology.[28]

Dialectical behavior therapy (DBT) was developed as a treatment for borderline personality disorder, but has some evidence for reducing self-injury.[29] DBT combines elements of cognitive behavior therapy with Zen mindfulness practices. Within DBT, clients practice mindfulness, learn how to tolerate distress, work on interpersonal relationships, and develop skills for emotion regulation.[19] These skills are often taught in a group format, supplemented by one-on-one therapy to help the client apply these skills in their life. Although typically focused on the individual, the program has been adapted to include families. The family program aims to educate family members about borderline personality disorder, work with family members to promote a validating family environment, and address emotion regulation and interpersonal skills for all family members.[30]

Mentalization-based therapy was developed as a way to improve mentalization ability, particularly for individuals with borderline personality disorder.[31] The goal is to help clients better understand their own thoughts and feelings, as well as those of others. Mentalization-based therapy has evidenced reductions in self-harm (broadly defined) among adolescents,[32] although among treatment-seeking adults it may not be superior to DBT.[33] There have also been calls to include a deliberate focus on mentalization in family therapy.[34] Self-reflecting parenting programs, developed to help parents develop mentalization in their children, show some promise.[35] Although a handful of studies show promising results for mentalization-based therapies, much more research is needed to determine whether they can effectively reduce self-injury.

Drawing on narrative therapy, letter writing has also been suggested as a part of family therapy for self-injury.[36] Here, letters might include:

1. families working together to write to an externalized form of self-injury to request it loosen its grip on the client (e.g., Dear Fred, we understand you are helping our daughter cope with her depression right now, but could you please give her a bit of a break so she can try other ways to cope?)

2. a client writing a letter to themselves in the present (e.g., Dear Sophie, I'm sorry to hear you are feeling down, but know that you have a great family to support you in this difficult time)
3. the family writing from the future (Dear Tarek, I remember when you were going through that really tough time. I'm so proud to see how far you have come and all that you have achieved)
4. the therapist writing to the family to acknowledge their efforts (e.g., Dear family, Knowing your son is struggling at the moment can be really hard. I see how hard you are working together as a family to help him, and that you are supporting him the best you can).

Emotionally focused family therapy is a third family therapy proposed to treat self-injury.[37] Emotionally focused family therapy also has its roots in the attachment relationship, but additionally has a focus on emotion within the family context. We are not aware of empirical work supporting any of these approaches with self-injury, but given the significant role of families in the course of self-injury, healing family relationships is bound to be important.

IMPACT ON FAMILIES

Inasmuch as self-injury has an impact on the person engaging in the behavior, it also has a significant impact on families and caregivers. Caregivers are often unaware their child self-injures, and can react with shock, worry, guilt, shame, and helplessness. Caregivers may thus question their parenting abilities and wonder how they "missed" that their child was in such pain. In addition to anxiety and mental health concerns, caregivers report physical effects of knowing their child self-injures, including heart palpitations, sleeplessness, weight loss, and feeling physically ill.[38] This *parental secondary stress* can be objective strain (e.g., financial hardship, disrupted routines), subjective strain (e.g., feeling resentful or embarrassed), or subjective internalized strain (e.g., guilt, worry[39]). The extent of this strain is related to how much the caregiver feels responsible for the self-injury and the severity of the self-injury itself. Parents of adolescents who self-injure report greater judgment and less compassion for both themselves and their child, and report less optimism for the future.[40]

Although all caregiver reactions are valid, and often reflect concern for the young person, unfortunately they can have detrimental effects on the individual who is self-injuring, and other family members. Some parents can be dismissive of self-injury, viewing it is a phase or as attention seeking. Concerned parents may also overmonitor their child, removing implements that could be used to self-injure, checking social media, and limiting social interactions. Neither reaction is helpful for the young person who self-injures. Dismissing the behavior invalidates the experience of the young person, while hypervigilance risks the trusting relationship a caregiver may have with their child. Further, given that over controlling parenting is a risk factor for self-injury,[41] such actions may exacerbate self-injury risk.

The self-injury family distress cascade theory proposes a *complementary escalation* of responses on the part of both a young person who self-injures and their caregiver.[42] The authors of this model focus on adolescence as the time at which self-injury most often starts, and thus situate their theory within a developmental framework. Noting that the formation of a unique identity and search for autonomy are two key developmental milestones during adolescence, the authors propose that self-injury may be used as one way to demonstrate autonomy. Questioning and overcontrolling measures used by caregivers in response to self-injury threaten this autonomy and may lead the young person to increase efforts to hide the self-injury from caregivers. They note that, perhaps unconsciously, the adolescent who is in search of autonomy may push caregivers to restrict that autonomy; on the other hand, caregivers seek reassurance about the well-being of their child, which is perceived as invalidating or controlling by the young person.[42] This cycle has the potential to escalate, furthering risk of self-injury and exacerbating anxiety felt by caregivers. Further work with parent-child dyads is needed to explore the complex family dynamics, and how they may change once a caregiver becomes aware their child is self-injuring.

BEING SUPPORTIVE IN THE CONTEXT OF RECOVERY

One of the most important roles parents and caregivers can play is to simply be there to listen when their young person seeks support. Given the significant stigma associated with self-injury, and the need to maintain autonomy, young people may be reluctant to disclose their self-injury, or talk about it with family. Young people preferentially seek support from friends rather than turning to adults in their lives. When we asked young people what parents and caregivers could do to support someone who self-injures, they overwhelmingly said that parents could listen to their children (Table 9.1).[43] Some suggested bringing the whole family together to talk or that caregivers could help by seeking formal support for the person who self-injures. In line with this, young people highlighted the importance of the family environment, and bonding experiences, suggesting that caregivers organize family outings to spend time together. Finally, young people stressed that families play an important role in reducing stigma by responding appropriately and avoiding judgment. Young people are more likely to seek support from parents and caregivers if they anticipate being able to openly discuss their self-injury without judgment.[43]

Initial Conversations

Broaching the topic of self-injury with a young person can be difficult. Yet, how a parent or caregiver addresses the issue, and how they respond to the concerns of

Table 9.1. WHAT YOUNG PEOPLE THINK CAREGIVERS CAN DO TO SUPPORT INDIVIDUALS WHO SELF-INJURE.

Listen to Them	Referral to a Professional	Reduce Stigma	The Family Context
• Talk to their kids	• Contact someone who can help	• Don't look down on them	• Go on family outings
• Try and listen to their problems	• Make an appointment with a counselor	• Avoid judgment	• Make sure the child knows they are loved
• Have a chat with them	• Advise them to see the school counselor	• Don't get angry	• Avoid conflict in front of young people
• Ask them what is going on for them	• Go with them to a psychologist	• Don't assume the behavior is suicidal	• Involve children in things that make them feel good about themselves
• Allow young people to be honest about how they feel		• Try to be understanding	• Sign them up for activities they enjoy (e.g., dance, sport)

SOURCE: Adapted from: Berger, E., Hasking, P., & Martin, G. (2013). "Listen to them": Adolescents' views on helping young people who self-injure. *Journal of Adolescence, 36*, 935–945.

the young person in their lives, is critical to the outcomes for the young person. Dismissing the self-injury, overreacting, being judgmental, or getting angry are not helpful responses. These are likely to further distance the young person, encouraging secrecy and potentially increasing risk of self-injury. If a parent or caregiver suspects their child is engaging in self-injury, it is important they choose an appropriate time to approach the child. Choosing a time and a space that is quiet, safe, and free from distraction from other family members is critical. From here, it is advised that parents ask the young person openly about the self-injury. For example, if a caregiver has noticed signs of self-injury they might say:

> "I've noticed these marks on your arms. I know some people self-injure as a way to cope with stress. Is this something you have been doing?"

It is important to validate how the young person is feeling and recognize that they are struggling with something, using a *respectful curiosity*.[44] In this regard, a caregiver might say:

> "I'd like to understand what is going on for you and how self-injury helps. Can you help me understand?"

They might also be honest with their own feelings, which communicates concern for the young person's well-being:

> "To be honest, I am a little uncomfortable with this because I don't like to see you hurt."

Parents and caregivers can recognize that talking about self-injury may also be uncomfortable for the young person and they may struggle to express how they are feeling, or why self-injury seems to help. It is important not to push young people to talk if they do not want to. Caregivers can let young people know that when they are ready to talk, they will be there for the young person. They may also offer to set up an appointment with a psychologist or counselor, or work together to develop a safety plan (see Chapter 2) that might provide alternative options if the young person wants to stop or reduce their self-injury.

Parents or caregivers might be tempted to ask the young person to promise not to self-injure, or to remove access to tools someone might use to self-injure. However, these options are likely to be unhelpful for a number of reasons. First, the young person is likely to be using self-injury as a coping strategy. It might seem counterintuitive, but self-injury does work to reduce distress—at least in the short term. Some people use self-injury to *feel something*, when they feel empty or depressed. Asking someone to stop using an effective coping strategy does not leave them with many options for coping with intense or unwanted emotions. Second, asking someone not to self-injure, or removing tools, decreases autonomy for the young person and may prompt secrecy rather than open communication. If the young person continues to self-injure they are more likely to hide it and not seek support. As noted above, overmonitoring or overcontrolling parenting can increase risk of self-injury. Third, individuals who self-injure need to function in a world that contains implements that might be used to self-injure. One aspect of working on reducing self-injury is resisting urges to self-injure, which may be prompted by seeing such tools. Taking the person-centered approach we advocate throughout this book, it is important that the young person is involved in decisions about how their self-injury is addressed and that they are able to voice their experiences without fear of judgment or panic on behalf of caregivers.

Ongoing Conversations

While a lot of attention has been paid to how to start a conversation about self-injury, there has been less recognition of the fact that, for families in which someone self-injures, this is likely to be an ongoing conversation. Parents and caregivers should know that it is okay to check in and see how the young person is doing—without pressuring them to talk if they do not want to or are not quite ready. If they have developed a safety plan together, they might review this to see if it is meeting the individual's needs or if it needs to be modified.

In line with a person-centered approach, caregivers should be mindful to not simply focus on the self-injury or allow it to define their relationship with their child. Although the young person may be struggling to cope with their emotions, they likely have several strengths that can be acknowledged and praised. Always focusing on the self-injury risks reducing the young person to this one behavior, rather than recognizing that it is just one form of coping that works for them right now. Throughout the recovery process, caregivers and families can reward the young person for small changes, like doing more housework, or getting on better with siblings, even if the self-injury is ongoing.

It is also important that parents and caregivers do not change normal routines or try to "protect" the young person by removing responsibilities the young person normally has (e.g., reasonable housework). Tiptoeing around the issue or "walking on eggshells" will create an atmosphere of anxiety within the family, and is not conducive to open and honest conversations. Although parents and caregivers may find it difficult or uncomfortable to know their child is self-injuring, parents have also told us that the experience brought them closer as a family, allowed them to get to know their child better, and opened opportunities for better communication (Table 9.2).[38]

Talking With Other Family Members

While self-injury clearly has an impact on the individual engaging in it, and on parents and caregivers, it also has an impact on siblings and the family dynamic. Parents and caregivers report changes in the family dynamic as a result of focusing attention on the child who self-injures.[38] This shift is also felt by siblings. In one study, siblings of young girls who self-injured felt their sister's self-injury determined the whole family life, and found family life distressing.[45] They felt they

Table 9.2. STRATEGIES FOR FAMILIES TO USE AND AVOID WHEN SUPPORTING
A CHILD WHO SELF-INJURES.

Helpful Strategies

- Find support for yourself (ideally through informal networks and professional support)
- Be clear about your expectations for your child about participating in family life and other activities
- Be collaborative and include your child in choices wherever possible (e.g., therapist, house rules, technology use)
- Acknowledge/Validate your son/daughter's pain/upset but remain calm throughout
- Choose times and places for hard conversations to maximize comfort and minimize distraction
- Keep lines of communication as open as possible
- Know that as much as you feel your son/daughter's upset/pain it is more helpful to your child to separate yourself from his/her feelings in order to stay calm in the face of their intensity
- Learn about self-injury and emotion/emotion regulation
- Ask your child open, honest questions—questions without an agenda asked in a sincere and respectful way
- Model healthy coping strategies
- Understand and respect your child's readiness to change
- Help your child identify and reinforce successes
- Respect your child's wishes concerning sharing his or her self-injury with extended family, friends, or school
- Seek therapeutic support for you and for your family. Self-injury can cause family division; it helps for everyone to feel heard and understood
- Recognize that self-injury serves a purpose; knowing about how it helps and what to expect in recovery can be helpful

Unhelpful Strategies

- Blaming them for their self-injury
- Blaming yourself for your child's self-injury
- Getting caught up in their intense emotions and moods
- Taking sides with different family members about what is "right to do"
- Engaging in unnecessary power struggles (limit unilateral decisions and work for shared agreements wherever possible)
- Imposing a set of new "lock down" controls (e.g., monitoring whereabouts, requiring constant connection, limiting mobility)
- Unnecessary punishments and ultimatums
- Forcing conversation or requiring constant check-ins about self-injury or emotions
- Tiptoeing around the situation or setting reasonable expectations out of fear that you'll cause self-injury to happen.
- Taking doors off hinges and removing all possible self-injury implements from your home
- Insisting that your child cover old scars
- Removing reasonable family expectations (e.g., washing the dishes) as a way to "smoothing out" your child's emotional life
- Regularly jumping in to "fix" situations you think may trigger your child

SOURCE: Developed by the International Consortium on Self-injury in Educational Settings (used with permission).

did not get enough of their parents' attention, that there was felt sibling rivalry, and that parents favored the sibling who self-injured, by reducing limits set on them. Siblings also reported that their sister spoke to them about their self-injury, which they perceived as helpful for their sister, but distressing for themselves.

In addition to minimizing family disruption or being overprotective of the young person who is self-injuring, as outlined above, parents and caregivers can talk with siblings and other family members to help them better understand self-injury. Of course, this should always be done with the consent of the young person, and may involve the young person in the conversations. Parents and caregivers can educate siblings about self-injury and what function it serves for their brother or sister. However, given the potential for detailed discussion about self-injury to give rise to socialization effects (see Chapter 6), the focus should not be on the means of self-injury. Instead, siblings could be informed that self-injury is just one way their sibling is coping with whatever is going on for the right now. Parents and caregivers might like to talk about other ways the sibling(s) copes when they are upset or distressed to encourage, and reinforce, alternative coping strategies. Parents and caregivers can also acknowledge that self-injury might be confusing for siblings, and that they might feel the young person is getting all the attention. Above all, they can reassure siblings that they are loved, and are here for them if there are any issues—related to self-injury or not—that they would like to discuss.

CONCLUSION

Family environments are complex, and no two are alike. Some family environments might increase risk of self-injury, or self-injury might be used to help cope with a stressful or hostile family environment. Conversely, supportive family environments can be protective against self-injury. When a young person self-injures this can have a significant impact on families, and family dynamics. Parents and caregivers play a critical role in talking openly about self-injury with their young person, and in supporting siblings. Taking a person-centered approach, and adopting a respectful curiosity in these conversations, will allow the young person to feel more comfortable disclosing their self-injury and facilitate support seeking within the family system.

Clinical Approaches for Self-Injury

Assessment and Intervention

Typically, when working with individuals who self-injure, clinicians have drawn on a variety of techniques in the context of assessment in tandem with evidence-informed intervention strategies. Collectively, these are intended to work with clients with the aim of reducing (and eventually stopping) self-injury and thus to increase their overall well-being. The current chapter therefore covers what is generally recommended for the assessment of self-injury. This is followed by a general overview of the research-informed approaches typically used in intervention settings; we also bring attention to approaches receiving less empirical attention and flag those approaches generally not recommended in the field. This collective information is likely relevant to a broad range of clinicians and trainees who may, during the course of their work, interact with and support individuals who self-injure. We end the chapter by articulating how these approaches, while no doubt useful in many cases, can be augmented by incorporating a person-centered and strengths-based approach to foster recovery, which is unpacked further in the next chapter.

THE IMPORT OF RAPPORT

A basic tenet of effective clinical work is building and maintaining a strong therapeutic and collaborative alliance with a client. In the context of self-injury, establishing a good rapport is critical to obtaining insight into an individual's experience and, in turn, informing and guiding case conceptualization (i.e., a working but flexible understanding about what may account for a client's self-injury). Assessment thus sets the stage for a plan to work with an individual toward recovery. The importance of rapport cannot be overstated when working with individuals who self-injure. As discussed throughout Chapter 4, self-injury is widely stigmatized; thus, many individuals will have experienced negative interpersonal reactions about self-injury in the past or will anticipate such reactions, even when they have not directly happened to them. As a result, all past experiences along with any trepidation or concern about how people will respond to one's disclosure of self-injury will invariably be brought to clinical settings. The clinician working with a person who engages in self-injury must therefore be cognizant of this. Equally important, though, is awareness of one's own reactions to and views about both self-injury and individuals who self-injure. Failure to have this awareness is likely a recipe for weak and ineffective rapport and correspondingly, low motivation on the part of the client to engage in the therapeutic process.

To help foster a strong alliance with people who self-injure, several techniques have been recommended.[1-3] As noted by Barent Walsh, a renowned expert and clinician in the field, a "low-key, dispassionate demeanor" (p. 84) is essential in this regard.[3] This approach communicates that one is comfortable talking about self-injury and will do so devoid of judgment. Thus, the individual is accepted and their experience with self-injury is empathically validated. Unsurprisingly, certain means of responding can be ineffective, and in some cases quite harmful. For instance, an interactive style that communicates judgment (e.g., conveying disappointment or disapproval regarding a client's self-injury) will tell the individual they are doing something wrong. Approaches that involve a high degree of interest in self-injury are also not advised. Indeed, excessive interest in an individual's self-injury can be disconcerting and lead to a client wondering if the clinician is interested in other parts of their experience (e.g., factors that contribute to self-injury, concerns about disclosing self-injury to people in their lives). Finally, it is important to avoid effusive expressions of support as they can inadvertently reinforce or encourage self-injury engagement (e.g., an individual may come to believe that the only way to get such a response is through self-injury). Hence, a calm, low-key, but nonetheless compassionate demeanor offers a balanced means to talk about self-injury and develop good rapport. Coupled with this, it is recommended that the clinician conducting the assessment adopt a *respectful curiosity*,[1-6] which was highlighted in Chapter 2. This approach is particularly effective as it positions the clinician as learning from the individual about their own unique experiences with self-injury.[1-3,5,6]

ASSESSING SELF-INJURY

As rapport is built with an individual, clinicians are typically interested in understanding key areas about the client's experience with self-injury. Indeed, knowing about one's history of self-injury is conducive to identifying how to best support the client in reducing self-injury. Given the complexity of self-injury and people's experiences, there are several considerations in this regard. This typically includes understanding when an individual started to self-injure (age at onset), how one has self-injured (i.e., method/s), the frequency of their self-injury including its recency, the extent to which one has previously sought both medical and psychological services for self-injury, among other considerations (e.g., if someone has a main form of self-injury).

Understanding Why Individuals Self-Injure

In concert with the above, central to any assessment is ascertainment of why someone self-injures. A first step in understanding why someone self-injures is having a knowledge base about self-injury, including the reasons people self-injure (see Chapter 1). Outside of this, understanding the contexts in which one self-injures, including the many factors that can precede or provoke self-injury is critical. Therefore, attention to environmental, cognitive, affective, behavioral, and biological considerations can go a long way.[1-3,5,6] Table 10.1 presents examples of these considerations.

Table 10.1. CONSIDERATIONS FOR THE CONTEXT OF SELF-INJURY.

Context	Example Considerations
Environment	• Life events (e.g., arguments, setbacks, job loss, academic failure) • Social context of self-injury (e.g., being alone versus with a friend) • Broader contexts in which self-injury occurs (e.g., school, home, online) • Much like contexts in which self-injury occurs, it would also be important to identify those in which it does not
Cognition & Imagery	• Thoughts about oneself (e.g., I'm worthless, I hate myself) • Thoughts about self-injury (e.g., I can't resist my urges; I need to cut; I can't live without self-injury) • Thoughts about the world (e.g., life is unfair) • Thoughts about others (e.g., no one loves me, I have no support) • Images that one has preceding self-injury (e.g., of feeling trapped, alone) • Much like environmental contexts, attention should also be paid to the kinds of thoughts and imagery in which self-injury does not occur
Emotion	• Emotional states (shame, anger, distress, anxiety, sadness) • Attention to emotions that precede (e.g., distress) and proceed self-injury (e.g., relief • People's experience of emotions (e.g., intensity, frequency of particular emotions) • As with the prior domains, attention should also be paid to the kinds of emotional experiences in which self-injury does not occur
Behavioral	• Whether self-injury occurs alongside other behaviors such as substance use other potentially risky behaviors • As with the prior domains, attention should also be paid to the kinds of behavioral contexts in which self-injury does not occur
Biological	• Understanding factors which may impact coping and mood, such as insomnia, fatigue, illness, thyroid abnormalities

The use of a functional assessment has widely been noted as a useful approach to understand an individual's experience with self-injury and thus what may contribute to self-injury engagement.[1-3,5-7] Adopting this approach can help to identify many of the factors noted in Table 10.1 that have relevance to a person's experience with self-injury. More specifically, a functional assessment represents a collaborative enterprise in which a clinician works with a client to identify the triggers or antecedents (e.g., where one was, what one was thinking and feeling) preceding self-injury urges, whether self-injury was enacted in response to those urges (to determine whether urges were resisted or not acted upon), and what transpired after self-injury (e.g., changes in one's affect).

Using a functional assessment not only helps a clinician to identify what may be contributing to an individuals' self-injury and why it may be used recurrently but also can be useful for the individual, themselves. Indeed, it is not uncommon for people with lived experience of self-injury to report difficulty knowing what brings on their self-injury and thus why they do it. By breaking down the situations that have led to self-injury through a functional assessment, individuals may be better positioned to understand some of their personal triggers.

To facilitate this, the use of "chaining" or chain analysis from dialectical behavior therapy[8,9] may be beneficial. Here, the clinician asks more precise and temporally oriented questions to better understand what led to self-injury for an individual. For example, if an individual is unclear about what might have led to self-injury, a clinician might ask pointed questions that "walk through" the events that preceded self-injury (e.g., *Can you tell me where you were at the time? What happened after that?*)

Using chain analysis can help the clinician to understand not just the environmental context (e.g., argument with a partner) but also some of the more specific factors that led a client to self-injure, including specific thoughts (e.g., thinking this always happens, thinking the relationship may end) and feelings (e.g., feeling alone, a build-up of hurt). By engaging in this kind of process, a client may also develop a deeper understanding of the ways that environments or contexts contribute to their thoughts and feelings that may, in turn, contribute to urges to self-injure. By knowing what these factors are, both the clinician and client will be better positioned to implement strategies to use in the face of these experiences (e.g., coping strategies to employ when one notices a build-up of emotional hurt and that can ideally avoid a continued build-up that results in self-injury).

When first using a functional assessment, it is not uncommon to focus on the most recent time during which an individual has self-injured. This has the benefit of narrowing to a specific point in time but also one that is likely easier to recall. From here, functional assessments can be used in subsequent meetings between an individual and clinician as well as by individuals between appointments. As such, individuals may be asked to complete a short form or table between sessions as a means of monitoring self-injury and any changes that occur. For example, diary cards can be used to help an individual to track the times when self-injury occurs between sessions and thus to gain insight into why one self-injures.

Assessing Underlying and Co-Occurring Adversities

While it is certainly important to understand the proximal factors involved in one's engagement in self-injury through approaches such as a functional assessment, bearing in mind broader contextual factors is also key. Accordingly, it is recommended that attention be paid to some of the co-occurring and underlying factors that may be involved in one's self-injury experience. Thus, when conducting assessment in the context of self-injury, it would be important to keep in mind some of the mental health difficulties, life events, and co-occurring mental illnesses that are outlined in Chapter 1. From here and depending on the extent to which various factors are germane to one's experience, these considerations ought to be factored into the subsequent therapeutic approaches used. For example, if an individual has been experiencing major depression, addressing their depression alongside self-injury would be important.

Suicide Risk

Given the relation between self-injury and suicide described in Chapter 2, consideration of suicide risk is essential when working with individuals who engage in self-injury. With that said, avoiding assumptions (i.e., that one is at suicide risk by virtue of having self-injured) is also key. In this way, it is recommended that clinicians working with individuals with lived experience of self-injury inquire about suicide and to consider the aspect of suicide risk as they continue working with the individual. Indeed, as the course of self-injury may change with time, so too might one's risk for suicide. Because of this, it is imperative that any clinician working with individuals who self-injure be trained in and have efficacy in conducting a suicide risk assessment and safety planning.

INTERVENTION

We now turn to an overview of the different therapeutic approaches that are most often used in the context of intervention for self-injury. Although the evidence for these approaches is presented a bit later in the chapter, it should be mentioned that there is currently no single empirically supported treatment for self-injury. There are likely several reasons for this. First, as described in Chapter 2, there has been definitional inconsistency with respect to self-injury. If different studies use different definitions for self-injury, it is difficult to compare findings across studies. In line with this, some studies exclusively center on self-injury whereas others examine broader self-harm and thus consider self-injury and suicidal behavior together. Another issue is that many of the earlier studies in the field focused on groups with borderline personality disorder; thus, findings may not be generalizable to people who self-injure who do not meet these diagnostic criteria.

Beyond this, there are methodological considerations such as a small number of studies using randomized-control trials, studies relying on smaller sample sizes, not always having a control group, among other concerns (e.g., attrition, lack of long-term outcome assessment). Consequently, more research is needed in the area of intervention.

Although there is not yet an empirically supported intervention for self-injury, this is not the same as saying that treatments do not work. To the contrary, many people benefit from working with mental health professionals to address self-injury. It is more that the research needed to empirically validate a treatment is in its earlier stages, underscoring the need for more work in this area. Accordingly, we can view the approaches addressed next as *research-informed*. That is, they are suggested for use in the context of self-injury given some evidence that they may work to reduce self-injury in particular populations as well as research pointing to their utility for addressing concerns (e.g., coping difficulties) known to underlie self-injury. Among the approaches discussed in this regard are cognitive behavior therapy, dialectical behavior therapy, family-based therapy (specific to working with youth who self-injure), and motivational interviewing. After introducing what these involve, we summarize some of the evidence for them. From here, we mention other approaches flagged as showing promise for reducing self-injury. We then bring attention to approaches that are advised against in treatment contexts. Please refer to Box 10.1 for a snapshot of psychological approaches used for self-injury, including those not recommended.

Box 10.1.

OVERVIEW OF PSYCHOLOGICAL APPROACHES.

PSYCHOLOGICAL APPROACHES TYPICALLY USED IN THE CONTEXT OF
SELF-INJURY TREATMENT.

Generally recommended approaches	Cognitive Behavior Therapy Dialectical Behavior Therapy Family-Based Therapy Motivational Interviewing
Other approaches with some empirical support	Emotion Regulation Therapy Interpersonal Psychotherapy
Implicated but needs empirical support	Compassion Focused Therapy
Not recommended	No Harm Contracts Replacement Behaviors

Cognitive Behavior Therapy

As noted earlier in the current chapter, different ways of thinking may have relevance in the context of one's self-injury engagement. It should therefore be of little surprise that therapeutic approaches that directly target specific thoughts or cognitive styles, have been highlighted as relevant in intervention for self-injury.[2,3,5,6,10,11] From a cognitive behavior therapy standpoint, self-injury would be conceptualized as resulting from what are referred to as "maladaptive thoughts" or "cognitive distortions" (e.g., *I am a bad person, self-injury is the only way to cope*).[2,3,10,11] Thus, having these thoughts would be seen as contributing to difficulty with regulating emotion or problem-solving, which, in turn, contributes to self-injury engagement.

Cognitive behavior therapy is used to help an individual to reduce their engagement in self-injury by challenging and modifying their "distorted" way of thinking. This might involve using thought records and other approaches (e.g., Socratic questioning) to identify relevant thoughts (e.g., *I'm stupid, I can't do anything*) that emerge in different contexts (e.g., after an academic setback), along with that situation's corresponding emotions (e.g., distress, shame) and resultant behaviors (e.g., self-injury). From here, individuals would work with a clinician to challenge the accuracy of these thoughts with the aim of developing new, "more adaptive" ways of thinking.

Given the interconnectedness of thoughts, emotions, and behavior, it would follow that by changing how one thinks in a given situation (e.g., *I had a setback but this doesn't mean I can't do anything*), there should be corresponding changes in both emotion (e.g., less distress/shame, relief) and behavior (e.g., not self-injuring, calling a friend instead). In this way, the use of cognitive behavior therapy would focus on ways of thinking with the overarching aim of fostering new ways of coping, communicating, and problem-solving. Although more research is needed to fully understand the effectiveness of cognitive behavior therapy to address self-injury, evidence from two reviews of the literature demonstrates that this approach has some utility in reducing self-injury by helping individuals challenge ways of thinking that contribute to self-injury engagement.[10,11]

Dialectical Behavior Therapy

Perhaps one of the most thought of interventions for self-injury is dialectical behavior therapy. In practice, this approach comprises both individual and group-based work; depending on the context; it may also involve phone skills training to use a phone and follow-up with a clinician on an as-needed basis.[9,12,13] Dialectical behavior therapy can be viewed as a form of cognitive therapy as it draws on the latter's principles but adds several approaches believed to help individuals better understand their emotional experiences; this includes how to cope with unwanted and especially intense or difficult emotions. Among these strategies are the promotion of distress tolerance (e.g., learning to sit with upsetting emotion), emotion regulation (e.g., coping skills), interpersonal effectiveness (e.g., active listening, assertiveness), and mindfulness skills. Due to the relevance of coping and emotion regulation in the context of self-injury (see Chapter 1), dialectical behavior therapy aims to augment how people respond to difficult emotions and thus how they respond to self-injury urges.

Although it may seem that this approach was specifically geared toward addressing self-injury, it was initially developed to treat borderline personality disorder. As discussed in Chapter 1, although self-injury is commonly engaged in by people who meet diagnostic criteria for borderline personality disorder, it is not circumscribed to this disorder. Nevertheless, the use of dialectical behavior therapy to specifically address self-injury makes sense given its focus on many of the concerns discussed in Chapter 1 that accompany self-injury. Along these lines, like cognitive behavior therapy, reviews of the treatment literature indicate that dialectical behavior therapy has some evidence to support its usefulness in helping individuals reduce the frequency of their self-injury engagement. This involves learning ways to accept and tolerate emotional pain, to respond to and manage urges to self-injure, and to navigate interpersonal difficulties.[10,11]

Family-Based Therapy

As adolescents represent a group that reports high rates of self-injury,[14,15] efforts have also focused on family-based approaches to treat self-injury. In some cases family involvement may be integrated into cognitive behavior therapy or dialectical behavior therapy, but family-based therapy is distinct in that the central focus of the intervention centers on the family and how they function.[10,11] Thus, the main goal is to address family functioning with the aim of reducing self-injury. Indeed, there are several reports that family functioning associates with self-injury engagement among youth (see Chapter 9).[16-18]

Therapeutically, various approaches can be used in the context of family-based therapy. These focus on the family-related factors thought to underlie a young person's self-injury and might include psychoeducation (to increase a family's understanding of self-injury), providing training in how a family communicates (e.g., how a family discusses emotions), and problem-solving (e.g., how to respond to or cope with different dynamics, intense emotion). In this way, these approaches work to enhance the relationships within the family context.[10,11] Similar to the approaches discussed thus far, family-based therapy has also garnered some empirical support for its utility in enhancing families' understanding of self-injury, how they communicate with one another, and how they navigate conflict and develop solutions to problems.[10]

Motivational Interviewing

It should come as little surprise that many individuals who engage in self-injury will report difficulty in stopping the behavior. In many cases, there may be reluctance to stop or ambivalence about the prospect of no longer self-injuring.[19–21] This makes sense. For example, if self-injury has become a main form of coping, individuals may not know of other ways to manage difficult situations; thus, the thought of letting go of self-injury may be quite daunting. As a result, emphasis has been placed on the role of increasing motivation to work toward stopping self-injury through motivational interviewing.[22]

Underpinning motivational interviewing are three foundational components: collaboration (i.e., working with an individual and honoring their experiences and views), evocation (i.e., working to build on a client's own resources to spur intrinsic motivation to change), and autonomy (i.e., acknowledging and encouraging an individual's capacity for self-direction throughout the therapeutic process). Accordingly, a main goal of adopting this approach for self-injury is to cultivate a person's motivation to work toward stopping self-injury and fostering their personal agency in this regard.[19] This is accomplished by drawing on a range of techniques (e.g., rolling with resistance, identifying pros/cons of change) that are tailored to the individual. Although there is limited evidence for the use of motivational interviewing in the context of self-injury intervention, it has been identified as a potentially useful way to help individuals develop confidence and motivation to work toward stopping the behavior.[19] Notably, it may offer usefulness both prior to and throughout the treatment process.[10,19]

Other Forms of Intervention

For the most part, the above approaches have received the most attention in the field. There are others, however, that warrant some discussion. For instance, interpersonal psychotherapy and problem-focused therapy have varying degrees of evidence in the context of self-injury.[6,10,11] Beyond treatments that stem from a single modality (e.g., cognitive behavior therapy) are those that blend together components from more than one. For example, emotion regulation group therapy,[23,24] which draws on components of dialectical behavior therapy and acceptance and commitment therapy, has been shown to reduce self-injury frequency among women with co-occurring symptoms of borderline personality disorder.[23–25] It may therefore have relevance to other groups who also engage in self-injury.

More recently, approaches such as compassion-focused therapy have been flagged as relevant in the treatment of self-injury.[26] Reasons for this come from research indicating that many individuals who engage in self-injury report higher levels of self-criticism (and even self-loathing), and that by being more compassionate toward oneself, one's self-criticism should diminish. In line with this, in the context of self-injury recovery, people have reported developing more compassion for themselves.[27,28]

Finally, with growing research focused on biological and physiological factors involved in self-injury,[29,30] it is important to comment on the use of medication. While more research is needed to inform best-practice guidelines, there is some evidence for the use of certain medications (e.g., selective serotonin reuptake inhibitors, atypical antipsychotics, naltrexone) to reduce self-injury.[11] However, the use of medication would normally occur alongside psychological approaches versus being used as a standalone treatment.[11]

APPROACHES NOT RECOMMENDED

Before concluding the chapter, it is important for readers to be aware of the kinds of treatment approaches that are not advised due to either their ineffectiveness or potential for harm. One such approach used with more ubiquity in the past are "no-harm" agreements or contracts. These tend to involve an agreement between an individual and the clinician in which the individual agrees to not engage in self-injury as part of—and at times as a condition of—treatment. Using this kind of approach is bound to set an individual up for failure.[2,3,5,31] Indeed, as described in Chapter 11, recovery is a nonlinear process during which there are inevitable setbacks. Thus, expecting that one should be able to stop self-injury before beginning treatment represents an unrealistic expectation on the part of both the person who self-injures and the clinician. After all, if it were that easy to stop, the need for intervention would ostensibly be quite low. Rather than promote motivation to work on recovery, these approaches can instead provoke shame (e.g., if one self-injures after agreeing to not self-injure) and secrecy (e.g., fear and thus reluctance about disclosing self-injury if it happens). Ultimately, such outcomes are likely conducive to thwarting motivation to work toward recovery and weakening—if not fracturing—the therapeutic alliance.

Another approach that has generated some controversy in the field is the use of replacement behaviors. Here, acts intended to mimic or resemble self-injury are suggested for use in place of self-injury when urges arise. Examples include snapping rubber bands on one's wrist, using a red marker on one's skin, or holding ice-cubes for a period of time. In some cases, individuals may find these kinds of strategies useful; however, this is far from universal and there are concerns that using them does not address a person's underlying needs.[32] Although replacement strategies are used, and even endorsed as a part of the National Institute for Health and Clinical Excellence's (NICE) guidelines to treat broader self-harm[33] they are generally not advised for self-injury.[34,35] Bolstering this is recent research in which the views of people with lived experience were elicited. Here, it was found that the use of replacement behaviors and other strategies under the umbrella of harm reduction had short-term utility and were generally unhelpful in the reduction of self-injury engagement.[36] Instead these behaviors may suppress the emotional experience, which paradoxically increases distress and could lead to more severe self-injury. Further, these behaviors themselves could be used as a form of self-injury.

CONCLUSION

Central to any treatment approach for self-injury is first conducting an assessment. As noted early in the chapter, there are many considerations that need to be accounted for, including not only key domains of interest (e.g., frequency of self-injury, reasons for self-injury) but also how one conducts the assessment (e.g., using a low-key compassionate demeanor) to build rapport with an individual client. Indeed, without attention to these considerations, rapport is likely to be weak, which compromises how well a clinician can understand an individual's experience.[1-3] Informed by a comprehensive assessment, clinicians can then draw on an array of approaches that address many of the difficulties that can play a role in self-injury engagement.

Although more research is certainly needed, there are several approaches that appear to have some evidence for their usefulness in helping individuals reduce the frequency of their self-injury.[10,11] Indeed, many individuals who have lived experience have benefited from these approaches. At the same time, many of the approaches outlined in this chapter seem to place most emphasis on reducing self-injury. On the one hand, this is an understandable goal and, from a research standpoint, represents a clear measurable outcome; on the other hand, we argue that narrowing or at least placing too much emphasis on the behavior may inadvertently ignore other salient parts of a person's experience.

Of course, we recognize that in therapeutic settings, most clinicians will not solely focus on the cessation of self-injury and will instead pay attention to underlying adversities that play contributory roles to one's self-injury (e.g., depression, eating disorders, difficulty coping) and thus an individual's overall well-being. Nevertheless, we contend that even when using the approaches outlined in this chapter, core features of people's lived experience of recovery may be missed. For example, as mentioned in our person-centered recovery framework in the next chapter, individuals often have concerns about scarring and disclosing self-injury to others. Thus, incorporating these concerns in any approach is apt to be important as it works toward ensuring that all their needs are met.

Many of the approaches discussed here are also grounded in deficit-based literatures. For example, in the context of cognitive behavior therapy, one would be viewed as having maladaptive or distorted thinking; and, in a dialectical behavior therapy context, one may be viewed as lacking interpersonal or distress tolerance skills. This is not to say people do not benefit from learning new strategies in these. They very often do. Rather, if the primary focus lies on what one does not have, the opportunity to harness the inherent strengths of people with lived experience may be missed. In the next chapter we therefore discuss approaches that can be used when working with individuals who self-injure given their overt emphasis on strengths and resilience building.

Self-Injury Recovery

A Person-Centered Framework

As discussed in prior chapters, the language used when discussing self-injury and the overall experience of self-injury is a paramount consideration. The same applies when considering the topic of recovery in the context of self-injury. The term "recovery" is used widely by individuals with lived experience of self-injury when describing their self-injury experiences.[1-3] Indeed, many people with lived experience view the term "recovery" as appropriate and acceptable, unlike other terms (e.g., "maladaptive coping strategy"; "self-injurer").[4-6] Outside of lived experience contexts, mention of recovery is also pervasive in both research and clinical literatures.[3,7-10] Accordingly, we have elected to use "recovery" as a referent throughout this chapter, and in others. Despite the commonness of the term's use, we are cognizant that the term "recovery" may not fit for all individuals with lived experience and that some people will elect to use different terms and framings when referring to their experience.

With this in mind, the primary aim of this chapter is to present a novel, person-centered framework with which to conceptualize self-injury recovery—one that is grounded in lived experience perspectives.[11,12] This model departs from many other framings of self-injury recovery. We believe, however, that such a model is not only appropriate but also critical to advancing the field and as discussed in Chapter 12, facilitating positive outcomes among people with lived experience of self-injury. Before discussing this new model, however, it is important to first discuss alternate frameworks that could be used to understand recovery and those that have been historically applied in this regard.

ALTERNATE RECOVERY FRAMEWORKS

Psychiatric Approach to Recovery

Despite the widespread nature of its use, the concept of recovery may seem ill-suited when considered in the context of self-injury. The term recovery has traditionally been used in medical and clinical settings in reference to particular diseases or ailments. In contrast, self-injury, while sometimes occurring in the context of mental illness, is fundamentally a behavior. Nevertheless, given this association, self-injury is clinically germane and there has been much debate about whether it ought to be considered a standalone mental disorder.[13] Commensurate with this, as indicated in Chapter 1, self-injury has been included in Section 3 of the *Diagnostic and Statistical Manual* (5th ed.; DSM-5) as a condition warranting further consideration; here, it is referred to as Non-Suicidal Self-injury (NSSI) Disorder.

With growing research in this area, it seems likely that NSSI Disorder will be formally incorporated in a future revision of DSM. Should this occur, a psychiatric approach to recovery could very well be adopted. Therefore, much like other mental disorders for which such a framing may be used, people who self-injure would be considered "recovered" when they no longer meet diagnostic criteria for NSSI Disorder. Taking a closer look at the proposed criteria for NSSI Disorder at the time of this writing, this would mean that people have: (a) not self-injured on more than 5 days in the prior 12 -months; (b) have not self-injured for a purpose (e.g., to self-punish); (c) no longer have urges or preoccupations about self-injury; and (d) no longer experience impairment or interference in their lives resulting from self-injury (e.g., self-injury no longer impacting people's social lives).[14]

Interestingly, the bulk of research attention in this area has been paid to the first criterion, which pertains to frequency of the behavior (i.e., self-injury has occurred on 5 days or more in the past 12 months).[15] Intentional or not, this focus on frequency implies that reducing (and perhaps eliminating) self-injury is a central aim of intervention. While this is understandable and such a goal likely aligns with the aims of many clinicians and individuals who self-injure, people with lived experience of self-injury have expressed concern that too much emphasis on frequency may inadvertently dismiss the various underlying factors contributing to self-injury (e.g., difficulty with coping, major depression, past trauma).[16] As discussed later in the chapter, people with lived experience describe a multitude of considerations (beyond cessation) as central in recovery.

Stages of Change Model

Beyond a psychiatric lens with which to view self-injury recovery, a commonly used framework is the transtheoretical model (also referred to as the stages of change model).[17] Fundamental to this model is that change in people's behavior transpires over time and that people shift through different stages as they work to no longer engage in a given behavior. Specifically, behavioral change translates to the ultimate cessation of the behavior of interest.

Overall, the transtheoretical model[17] is composed of five stages in which both behavioral and cognitive processes play a role in moving someone from one stage to the next. The stages of the model are Precontemplation (this is before individuals are ready to change and are thus not considering change in the next 6 months); Contemplation (when individuals intend to change in the next 6 months); Preparation (when people intend to take action in the next month); Action (when people are actively making effort to change); and Maintenance (when people have made behavioral changes that last for 6 months or longer). As individuals work through the model's stages, it is theorized that they develop self-efficacy to not act on urges that previously led to the behavior, which allows them to resist urges as they occur. Finally, within the transtheoretical model, a decisional balance is used in which the pros and cons of engaging (or not) in the behavior are weighed.[17]

There is some evidence that the transtheoretical model may offer some utility in the context of self-injury recovery.[18,19] Further, the transtheoretical model may have relevance in a recovery context given its explicit recognition that people can be ambivalent when it comes to stopping the behavior.[20] Congruent with this, it is common for individuals with lived experience to express uncertainty and ambivalence about stopping self-injury altogether, especially if it has been an effective coping strategy for them.[21,22] Another reason the transtheoretical model may have relevance is that people may have recurrences of the behavior in the context of recovery. Indeed, part of the model indicates that movement through the different recovery stages is recursive, and people may experience relapse.[17] Along these lines, acknowledgment that recovery might involve setbacks is a realistic, normative, and encouraging way to view recovery in that setbacks will not deter ongoing recovery efforts.

Although the transtheoretical model has garnered some support when understanding self-injury recovery,[18,19] its application to self-injury may be limited in that it does not capture the full complexity of self-injury recovery discussed by people with lived experience. For instance, the transtheoretical model suggests that individuals move through particular stages.[17] And, as one moves from one stage to the next, particular milestones must be met.[23] For example, in the final stage of the transtheoretical model (Maintenance), it is expected that people no longer engage in the behavior of interest for a 6-month period. Not only is this period of time arbitrary but not meeting this benchmark may be viewed as a lack of progress or even failure. Certainly, this kind of perspective is unhelpful as it can thwart future motivation to work on recovery.

Much like the psychiatric approach, much of the emphasis in the transtheoretical model is again placed on cessation of self-injury. While it is reasonable, indeed inevitable, to consider cessation of self-injury in the context of recovery, too much focus on this outcome can place unnecessary pressure on people who engage in self-injury. This, in turn, can leave people feeling they have not "recovered" regardless of elapsed time since one last self-injured.[9,21] Finally, as mentioned before, overemphasis on the frequency of self-injury detracts from the multitude of considerations people with lived experience express as highly salient in the context of their own recovery.[11,12] For these reasons, while both psychiatric and transtheoretical model approaches have varying degrees of utility, they may be limited in scope and relevance to people's lived experience.[12]

Research on Self-Injury Recovery

In addition to understanding the frameworks that may have applicability to self-injury recovery, the research approaches that have been used in this context also deserve discussion. A review of the studies published to date indicates that both quantitative and qualitative methods have been used. Regarding the former, this has typically involved studies conducted with the aim of identifying how individuals who report no longer self-injuring differ from individuals who report recently self-injuring. To this end, researchers have sought to establish how variables believed to be central in recovery (e.g., emotion regulation) vary between these groups.[12] On the one hand, these approaches can be useful in that they can bring attention to factors that may be relevant to fostering recovery. On the other hand, examining how groups who do and no longer self-injure differ precludes our ability to draw conclusions about whether and how these differences play facilitative roles in recovery and whether recovery occurs because of these changes.[12] For example, it may be that people who have more resources in place (e.g., a support system, access to services) simply self-injure less often as time passes.

Outside of quantitative approaches, research on self-injury recovery has also been conducted qualitatively. Here, people with lived experience have typically been asked open-ended questions about their recovery experiences or their experiences shared in different contexts (e.g., online) have been examined for their content and meaning.[12] By virtue of using these approaches, insight have been obtained into the nature of people's recovery experiences, including what recovery means to them.[9,21] To this end, many individuals do not conceptualize recovery as just behavioral cessation.[9] Rather, they report ongoing thoughts and urges as well as ambivalence about completely stopping self-injury.[18,24] They also discuss various enduring effects of self-injury such as scarring,[9,25] stigma,[26] and disclosure[9,26] as well as the need to address underlying concerns such as underlying mental health difficulties.[9] When considered collectively, recovery from a lived experience vantage point is indeed multiplex in nature.

Final Notes

As presented so far, there are several ways that recovery can be and has been conceptualized. And, while some of these have demonstrated at least some utility and empirical support,[18,19] we argue that they are still not well-suited to understand the complexity of, and ultimately foster, self-injury recovery. Instead, we advocate for an approach that draws on both quantitative and qualitative research and, critically, places people's lived experience at the forefront—an approach that acknowledges the many and often intersecting factors that can contribute to self-injury alongside those that have salience in people's lives. Moreover, our model places emphasis on the capacity for people to build strength and find meaning in their own recovery experience. Thus, in what follows, we offer a person-centered and strengths-based framework that accounts for the totality of these considerations.

A PERSON-CENTERED RECOVERY FRAMEWORK

Although self-injury cessation can be viewed within the context of the model, we intentionally adopt a multifaceted approach to conceptualize recovery to ensure that considerations beyond stopping the behavior are highlighted. Before discussing the model, it is important to address several key assumptions. First, we do not assume that recovery is the same for everyone. Indeed, a true person-centered model cannot be a one-shoe-fits-all approach. Rather, the model is deliberately flexible in nature. Hence, some components in the framework will have more salience for some people when compared to other individuals. Second, we do not consider recovery to unfold as a linear or stage-like process. Whereas other models assume that recovery is a stepwise progression from self-injuring to no longer self-injuring, we do not view recovery as comprising a particular sequence of steps. Relatedly, we do not believe that there is a specific timeframe by which recovery ought to occur (as might be the case in some of the aforementioned approaches).

Following the above, and as articulated *by* people with lived experience, we believe that recovery is and should be viewed as a nonlinear process.[9,11,12] In consonance with this, the process of recovery involves much more than cessation of self-injury. Moreover, we see this process as one in which people can develop inner strength, find meaning, and cultivate resilience along the way. This can occur, for example, by finding new ways to cope and relating to the self. With this in mind a core tenet of this model is that people have the capacity not only to stop self-injuring but also to identify and foster strengths as they navigate through their own recovery. In this way, the model we present below is a composition of several components: *Realistic Expectations and Setbacks*; *Normalizing Thoughts and Urges*; *Fostering Self-Efficacy*; *Identifying Strengths*; *Finding Alternatives*; *Addressing Underlying Adversities*; *Addressing and Accepting Scarring*; *Navigating Disclosures*; and *Self-acceptance and Self-compassion*. Our person-centered, strengths-based model is illustrated in Figure 11.1.

Realistic Expectations and Setbacks

In line with the basic premises of our model, we recognize that people with lived experience of self-injury will hold different views and expectations when it comes to their own recovery. As highlighted in prior research, even when there are similarities between people, self-injury recovery is nevertheless a unique experience for everyone.[9,21] It is therefore essential that we consider people's unique views about recovery and what they expect recovery to entail.[9] Doing so is critical not only to understanding how people approach recovery (e.g., with trepidation,

Ongoing, Nonlinear, & Individual Process

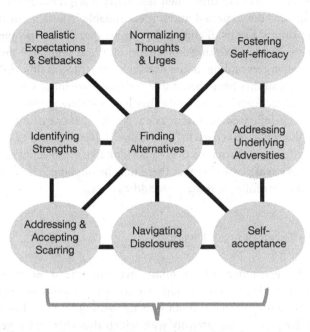

Fostering Resilience & Making Meaning

Figure 11.1. Person-centered recovery model.

with ambivalence) but also to fostering and sustaining motivation to work toward their own recovery.

Early on, it is important that people have expectations about recovery that are realistic in nature. Based on research conducted to date, some people will conceptualize recovery as all-or-nothing and, as such, equate recovery with the complete stoppage of self-injury as well as the end of self-injury thoughts and urges.[9,21] In many ways, these expectations make sense as they likely represent a desire to be "free" from self-injury. Yet, these views are also unrealistic; most (if not all) individuals will have at least some thoughts about self-injury in the future. Despite them being understandable, the overarching concern with more absolute views about recovery is that, if held, then a recurrence of self-injury or the presence of ongoing self-injury thoughts and urges may contribute to a sense of helplessness about recovery and thus thwart future recovery efforts.

Research that draws on people's lived experiences tells us that recovery invariably waxes and wanes.[9,11,12] That is, due to the nonlinearity of recovery, individuals will typically experience setbacks or instances when recovery does not unfold as one would like (e.g., recurrences of self-injury). Importantly, how these instances are framed (e.g., setbacks, hiccups, blips) ought to be tailored to the individual (e.g., someone might view the term "setbacks" as negative whereas someone else might prefer this term). It is also important to bear in mind that such instances can even occur after stretches of time when self-injury has not occurred.[9] This is not only commonplace but expected and understandable. Afterall, self-injury often represents a primary means of coping for people; therefore, if people encounter stressful life events while working on recovery, it makes sense that they may turn to self-injury when responding to this stress. Congruent with this, participants in some of our own studies have shared that "relapses" are indeed an expected and *normal* aspect of recovery.[9] Importantly, they have further expressed that should a recurrence of self-injury occur, this does not signify that one cannot recover, nor does it mean that a person is back to "square one." Given this, it is essential that re-alistic expectations about what recovery may look like are fostered early on—this includes the very real possibility that there may be ongoing self-injury thoughts and urges that never fully go away, as we address next.

Normalizing Thoughts and Urges

In addition to recurrences of self-injury over the course of recovery, many individuals will continue to have thoughts and even urges concerning self-injury. Oftentimes, these may persist without fully dissipating.[9,24] Yet, while this may be the case, the frequency and intensity with which thoughts and urges occur are bound to subside. Accordingly, we do not view that recovery ought to require a lack of self-injury thoughts and urges. As mentioned above, most people will con-tinue to think about self-injury from time to time, even if short-lived; similarly, they may very well have future urges to self-injure. Because of this, it is impor-tant for people with lived experience to recognize that thoughts and urges about self-injury may never fully go away.[11,12] Similar to recurrences of self-injury, the future presence of thoughts and urges does not connote that one has failed in their recovery efforts.

If individuals with lived experience come to know that they may have thoughts about self-injury ongoingly, they are likely to be much better prepared and positioned to not just begin working on recovery but to persist with it. Having realistic expectations about this is not limited to people who self-injure, however. Key supports in their lives (e.g., families, partners) as well as the possible health and mental health professionals who work with them also need to have (and pro-mote) realistic expectations. This is conducive to being able to offer support and encouragement in the event of any "setbacks." Moreover, knowing what recovery entails can also reduce the likelihood of them becoming disheartened in terms of the support they offer.

Fostering Self-Efficacy

Many people with lived experience report that over the course of recovery, they develop a sense that they can resist acting on urges to hurt themselves when they occur. Such self-efficacy is key for many people in their recovery experience. One part of this involves coming to recognize and accept that thoughts and urges to self-injure may occur ongoingly, as discussed above. Another part of fostering self-efficacy is therefore understanding that it may vary across time, contexts, and across situations.[27] For example, someone might find it easier to not act on an urge to self-injure when at work but then experience more difficulty in this regard when home alone at night.[28]

Although the corpus of evidence in this area is relatively new, there are several studies that support the role of self-efficacy having a role in recovery. As an example, researchers have demonstrated that changes in self-efficacy are linked to stopping self-injury engagement.[29,30] Indeed, one's efficacy to not act on an urge to self-injure has been shown to coincide with the time since one last injured, with greater self-efficacy associating with a longer time since self-injury engagement.[29,30] Data from ecological momentary assessment research has similarly supported the role that self-efficacy can play in safeguarding against self-injury engagement.[31]

Ultimately, it is important that people develop a sense that they can experience and accept self-injury thoughts and urges and that their presence does not mean they have to hurt themselves. This is especially important as building self-efficacy to resist urges can help to manage and resist future urges to self-injure[31] and thus propel recovery efforts. In tandem with this, it is also important that self-efficacy be fostered in terms of drawing on alternate means to avoid self-injury.[32] For example, developing a coping repertoire to employ when urges arise may be useful as one could turn to an array of strategies instead of self-injury.

Identifying Strengths

Arguably, much of the research on self-injury over the years has used a deficit-based framing to theorize about and study the behavior. A review of the literature offers many such examples. For instance, early writings on self-injury pointed to the behavior being the product of a "failure to resist impulses to harm one's body."[33] Theory offered to explain the emergence and repetition of self-injury similarly highlighted the role that a lack of emotional validation can play.[34] Likewise, there are many reports that people who self-injure have poor emotion regulation skills or deficits in this area.[35,36] Although just a fraction of the field's total number of examples, each seems to imply that people are lacking or do not have enough of something, which contributes to self-injury. As such, these "deficits" would be targeted in treatment and recovery. We are not meaning to convey that people who self-injure do not experience difficulty coping nor are we conveying that people with lived experience of self-injury would not benefit from learning new ways to cope. Rather, what seems to be missing from much of the conversation and writing on self-injury are the many strengths that so many people with lived experience of self-injury have. We believe that these strengths can be harnessed and used to help propel the recovery process.

There are myriad examples of strengths among people who self-injure. Among just some of these are the close relationships people may have, qualities such as creativity, resilience, compassion for others (and the self), cognitive flexibility, having a sense of meaning or purpose, academic success, or having hobbies they are passionate about. Of course, there are copious more. Even when people have difficulty identifying their strengths, all people who self-injure will experience moments during which they have been able to resist urges to self-injure. These moments are, themselves, indicative of the potential to develop self-efficacy in the face of urges to hurt oneself. In doing so, there is also an opportunity to reflect on what was different at that time compared to times when an urge led to self-injury. We therefore recommend that alongside working with individuals who self-injure, clinicians inquire about and assess a person's strengths, resources for coping, and who they may have as supports in their life. From here, these can be integrated into the work done with an individual and a person's strengths can be leveraged to promote self-efficacy to resist urges to self-injure and thus to identify alternatives to self-injury, discussed next.

Finding Alternatives

As mentioned earlier when discussing self-efficacy, a core part of recovery tends to involve finding ways to not act on urges to self-injure and instead engage in alternate behaviors that can meet the need(s) that self-injury has met in the past. In support of this are the voices of people with lived experience who express that finding alternatives is critical to recovery.[9,21] Much like having realistic expectations about what recovery may involve, it is also important that people with lived experience recognize that finding an alternative that works for them may not happen immediately. It can often take time as well as trying different approaches before identifying strategies that work for and resonate with them. In concert with this, finding an alternative to self-injury is not a one-shoe-fits all approach. What works for one person may not work for the next and vice versa. It is therefore important that people who are working on recovery know that finding alternatives is indeed a process—it may take time and effort before finding a set of strategies that are a good fit for them. However, by way of having this insight early on it can help to sustain motivation to continue working on recovery, especially if earlier attempts are not as effective as perhaps anticipated.

Addressing Underlying Adversities

As highlighted in Chapter 1, there are countless adversities that can contribute to self-injury. Indeed, self-injury does not occur in a vacuum and people with lived experience have expressed that addressing self-injury necessitates consideration to what may underlie it.[16] Thus, our model of recovery highlights the import of accounting for these factors and putting self-injury into a proper and holistic context.

This includes giving consideration to the various mental health difficulties and mental disorders that may contribute to engagement in self-injury. Additionally, it involves attention to traumatic events and other touchstone adverse experiences people may have lived through. Beyond these, however, are those experiences that have not routinely or sufficiently been considered when understanding what may lead to and maintain self-injury. For example, this might include experiences with stigma or prejudice that people have unfortunately encountered. Likewise, attention ought to be paid to systemic issues such as racism or lack of access to support that may play a role in people's lived experience. No two people who self-injure are completely alike and it is essential that a person-centered approach be used to fully appreciate and acknowledge the many factors that can play a role in one's experience of self-injury.

Addressing and Accepting Scarring

A small but growing body of research has brought needed attention to the role that scarring from self-injury can play. In contrast to most other forms of mental health difficulties, self-injury is ostensibly unique in that it can result in permanent visible markings. Based on some of the research on self-injury scarring to date, people with lived experience have reported feeling significant shame and anxiety due to having scars.[25,37] This is not a universal experience, however. Many people with lived experience of self-injury have also expressed that with time, they come to look at their scars with a sense of compassion for themselves and thus come to accept their scars. In some cases, scars can come to signify strength and resilience to overcome prior adversities.[25,38]

In a recovery context scars from self-injury can play a key role. Findings from our own work reveal that individuals with lived experience of self-injury see scars as impacting recovery in different ways.[9] For some people, having scars and the feelings associated with them (e.g., shame) made people's recovery process more difficult. For other individuals, however, scars were said to symbolize a sense of strength and resilience. Taken together with the above, it is clear the presence of scars from self-injury has considerable germaneness to people's experience of self-injury and its recovery.[11,12] Thus, while not everyone will have scars from self-injury and people who do will inevitably differ in how they view them, their consideration in a recovery context is essential. In the next chapter we address some of the practical implications of this.

Navigating Disclosures

As discussed elsewhere in this book, self-injury is far too often marred by stigma, which makes it very difficult for many people to share their experiences with others.[26,39] Nevertheless, disclosing one's self-injury experience to another is a common concern for many people[40] and the same applies in a recovery context.[11,12]

This may be relevant in the early part of one's recovery experience such as to initiate recovery as well as later in terms of augmenting recovery.[41] Disclosure can also be important for people well after they have self-injured and in cases when people may consider themselves to be "recovered." As an example, some people may find meaning in sharing their experience in relationships in which they feel safe and understood. As such, disclosure of self-injury warrants attention in our framework as it can play a key role in initiating and enhancing recovery and in obtaining support from other people in both a professional context and in people's personal lives.

Self-Acceptance and Self-Compassion

We recognize and appreciate that recovery will look different for each person. With that said, we contend that recovery is possible for everyone and that people with lived experience have the capacity to develop self-acceptance and find meaning through their unique recovery journey. While clearly easier said than done, this can happen as individuals embark on recovery with realistic expectations, acknowledgment of the nonlinearity of the recovery process, and with time, develop efficacy to respond to and cope with urges to self-injure in new ways, and address the different adversities that may have contributed to the onset and repetition of self-injury. Supporting this view are findings from research, which indicate that people report developing inner fortitude and resilience,[9] acceptance of scarring and themselves,[25] and self-compassion and acceptance over the course of their recovery experiences.[42] In this regard, individuals can find themselves more prepared and equipped to tackle future stressors and adversities.

IMPLICATIONS FOR THE MODEL
EMPIRICAL IMPLICATIONS

Although informed by prior research, our person-centered, strengths-based framework presented here and elsewhere[12] should be studied for its utility in future research. Due to its person-centered nature, and because not all components will have relevance for any one person, larger-scale projects may be needed to increase the chances that all components of the model can be taken into account. In doing so, it will also be important to explore the model across different samples. Examples include youth, emerging adults, community versus clinical populations, and groups from socioeconomically and socioculturally diverse backgrounds as there may be unique considerations (e.g., systemic adversities) that might otherwise go overlooked.

In addition to large-scale studies, and consistent with the view that recovery is not universal across all people, approaches that employ within-person analyses will be needed. The design of these approaches can therefore include qualitative research involving interviews, but importantly consideration should be given to research that accounts for changes over time, such as diary studies or ecological momentary assessment. In a similar manner, longitudinal studies can work to examine the manner by which the nonlinear nature of recovery unfolds and how components of the model change in their level of import over time. Finally, since recovery does not occur in a vacuum, understanding other perspectives of recovery is essential. While a person-centered framing of recovery has the most relevance to the person who self-injures, our framework implicates the role of others (e.g., in the context of disclosure), including professionals, partners, and families. By shedding light on how recovery is understood and what role people can play in this regard, we will be much better positioned to facilitate recovery and promote well-being for people with lived experience.

Practical Implications

Although a more comprehensive discussion of the practical implications of our recovery model is reserved for the next chapter, a few important items warrant brief discussion. We have noted throughout the chapter that people with lived experience see recovery as a composite of many (and often interrelated) factors. We do not assume that clinicians who work with individuals who self-injure only think about or focus on self-injury cessation in their work. Many of the clinicians we know and have spoken with conceptualize recovery as much more than behavioral cessation. With that said, this concern is sometimes held by people who self-injure.[16] Thus, we see that our framework can benefit clinicians in their work with people who self-injure. By drawing on this framework, clinicians will have a new way of thinking about recovery and the many considerations that people who self-injure have. Using our model as a backdrop and guide in clinical work can thus highlight areas to explore with a client and, upon determining which are salient to the individual, working to address them. In doing so, there is a greater likelihood that the considerations most relevant to an individual are woven into the fabric of clinical work, thereby increasing the probability for improved outcomes for the client.

SUMMARY

Self-injury recovery is not straightforward, and no two people who self-injure and embark on recovery will have completely analogous experiences. For these reasons, it is imperative that recovery be conceptualized with a person-centered lens that circumvents making assumptions about what recovery entails for any one individual and permits an appreciation of its diverse, complex, and multifarious nature. Indeed, the framework outlined in this chapter is informed by the very concerns that people with lived experience have expressed as key in the process of recovery.[9,11,12,21] Although this may, for some people, represent a paradigm shift in terms of how recovery is conceived, we believe that adopting this approach has implications for research and clinical work that are far-reaching. And most importantly, by using this framework in both research and clinical contexts, we argue that a more holistic and compassionate understanding of self-injury can be achieved—one that sets the stage for the facilitation of recovery, building of resilience, and fostering of well-being among people who self-injure.

Building Resilience Through Recovery

Building resilience does not mean an individual will no longer face adversity or be affected by it. Instead, resilience is about being able to effectively cope and adapt in the face of life's challenges, and times of significant stress. For individuals who self-injure, this is often their way of coping with emotional turmoil, stress, and adversity. By recognizing self-injury recovery as a multifaceted process we see there are several opportunities to build resilience, even if someone continues to engage in self-injury.

REALISTIC EXPECTATIONS

Self-injury recovery is not as simple as an individual deciding they no longer wish to self-injure and then stopping the behavior. Any efforts at behavior change are difficult (e.g., trying to exercise more, going to bed earlier, eating a healthier diet) and require weighing up the pros and cons of change, as well as a combination of planning, goals, motivation, self-efficacy, and practice.[1] There are almost always setbacks in the behavior change process and it is no different with changing self-injury. As should be apparent from the recovery framework outlined in Chapter 11, recovery is a nonlinear process that proceeds in different ways, and at a different pace, for each individual. For many, this may involve instances of self-injury along the way, although over time these may become less frequent and intense.

What Can We Do to Foster Realistic Expectations?

In a clinical setting, it is important for the clinician to have an open and honest conversation with the client about their treatment goals, recognizing that cessation of self-injury may not be an immediate goal for the client. If self-injury cessation is a goal, it is important that individuals know that setbacks are normal, and to be expected, so they do not feel they have failed for self-injuring. Likewise, families and clinicians need to be mindful that the recovery process is not a linear one, and appreciate that someone may continue to engage in self-injury throughout their recovery. This does not mean gains are not being made in other areas (e.g., improving self-efficacy, slowing adding alternative coping strategies to the repertoire), and families and clinicians should take care not to perpetuate any shame an individual may feel because of their ongoing self-injury.

How Do We Help People Bounce Back From Setbacks?

For some, resilience is conceptualized as the ability to "bounce back" from challenges. As such, resilience can be fostered in the way an individual approaches a setback or a slip in their self-injury recovery. In the alcohol dependence field, Marlatt and Gordon[2] make a distinction between a "lapse" and a "relapse." If an individual trying to abstain from alcohol has a drink this is considered a lapse, and it is how the individual responds to this lapse that determines whether they relapse into dependent drinking. Specifically, Marlatt and Gordon note that a combination of being in a high-risk or emotional situation, positive expectancies regarding the potential outcome of the behavior, lowered self-efficacy to resist the behavior, and a lack of alternative coping strategies increases the likelihood of a lapse. Once this lapse, or first drink, occurs individuals may encounter an "abstinence violation effect." This effect is a cognitive process that includes a sense of cognitive dissonance (e.g., experiencing guilt as a result of violating one's abstinence goal), and blaming oneself for the lapse. These cognitions can also be accompanied by a feeling of loss of control over the behavior. If an individual is able to counter their cognitive dissonance, by reframing the event (e.g., *"it's just one drink, that does not mean I am not on the path to recovery"*) this may lessen the chance of continued drinking and relapse. Conversely, the abstinence violation effect may be too strong to counter an individual's abstinence goal, with a sense of failure leading to thoughts such as *"well I've had one drink. I've blown it, I may as well keep drinking,"* which increases the chance of continued drinking.

Although we are in no way suggesting self-injury is an addiction, a similar process may be involved in self-injury setbacks, or instances of self-injury that occur during recovery. As such, clinicians and families can work with individuals to reframe instances of self-injury (see Table 12.1).

NORMALIZING THOUGHTS AND URGES

Thoughts of, and urges to, self-injure can persist long after an individual ceases to actively engage in the behavior. Again, this should be made clear to individuals who self-injure, early in the recovery process, to foster realistic recovery expectations, and to support individuals who may perceive that they are not recovering if these thoughts persist. Indeed, when we ask individuals how they will know they

Table 12.1. EXAMPLES OF REFRAMING INSTANCES OF SELF-INJURY.

Ways to reframe instances of self-injury when they occur during recovery
- It's just a one-off; this doesn't mean I will continue to self-injure
- I may still self-injure occasionally, but not as often as I used to
- This was a particularly overwhelming situation so it is not surprising I self-injured. I have a lot of other strategies I can use in less overwhelming situations
- This slip up does not mean I am a failure, I am still learning how to cope in other ways
- I have been really good at resisting urges to self-injure lately; this one slip up does not diminish that
- I self-injured this time, but I am starting to get some new coping strategies in my tool kit that I can use next time I feel overwhelmed
- I have a lot of strengths I can draw on to help me cope

have recovered they often say *"when I no longer have the urge to self-injure"* or *"when I don't think about it anymore."* As outlined in Chapter 11, this represents a fairly rigid conceptualization of recovery and one that is unlikely to be realistic. Significant gains in many areas of recovery, including in reducing engagement in self-injury, may be seen before thoughts and/or urges to self-injure desist.

So why would an individual experience ongoing thoughts or urges to self-injure? Although self-injury is associated with a range of adverse outcomes, there are also advantages to self-injuring.[3] For example, self-injury can provide immediate, although temporary, relief from emotional distress. Alternative coping strategies, on the other hand, can often require time and effort - and their benefits may be rather delayed as a result. Accordingly, it seems quite natural that an individual who has previously relied on self-injury to cope would want to turn to the behavior in times of heightened distress. At the same time however, an individual can hold the goal of wanting to stop self-injuring, and reducing the negative impacts such as feelings of guilt or permanent scarring. Holding both positive and negative views of self-injury can lead to a significant sense of ambivalence, wherein an individual simultaneously wants to self-injure, but also wants to reduce their self-injury.[4]

Acknowledging this ambivalence could go a long way to establishing rapport between a clinician and client, and pave the way for a more open and honest therapeutic relationship. Working within a motivational interviewing framework, conducting a decisional balance will allow a client and clinician the space to articulate competing goals.[5] In a decisional balance, the client and clinician work together to identify the costs and benefits of not changing the behavior, and the costs and benefits of changing the behavior (see Table 12.2). In the case of self-injury, acknowledging there are benefits to self-injury, but that the costs outweigh these, may help shift the motivation to reduce the behavior, and strengthen self-efficacy to resist thoughts and urges to self-injure. However, a decisional balance is best used either when attempting to identify ambivalence (i.e., not shifting the decision) or when more emphasis is placed on changing the behavior, or strengthening commitment to change (i.e., to guide a change conversation).[6,7]

Table 12.2. EXAMPLE OF A DECISIONAL BALANCE.

Benefits of Self-Injury	Costs of Self-Injury	Costs of Reducing Self-Injury	Benefits of Reducing Self-Injury
• Helps relieve tension	• Relief is only temporary	• Afraid I won't know how else to cope	• Long-term scarring will reduce
• ...	• Friends/family disapprove	• ...	• I'll learn a range of new coping strategies
	• It is painful		• I won't feel so out of control
	• It stops me doing things I want to do		• ...
	• I feel bad about myself when I self-injure		
	• ...		

BUILDING SELF-EFFICACY

Self-efficacy is a person's belief in their ability to perform a volitional behavior, and is one of the strongest predictors of whether someone engages in specific behaviors.[8,9] With regard to self-injury, self-efficacy can take many forms, including one's belief in the ability to deliberately hurt themselves and/or one's belief in the ability to resist urges to self-injure.[10] An inability to deliberately hurt oneself is a significant barrier to engaging in self-injury.[3] Similarly, self-efficacy to resist self-injury differentiates individuals with no self-injury history from those who have self-injured, and can differentiate people with a recent or past history of the behavior.[11] Further, a belief in the ability to resist self-injury can counter the risk conferred by expectations that self-injury will result in emotion regulation.[12] A growing body of research has demonstrated that people who self-injure tend to have lower general self-efficacy, including belief in the ability to cope, than individuals with no history of self-injury.[13-15] As an individual practices new coping strategies, self-efficacy to engage in alternative coping strategies will develop through the recovery process.

How Do We Develop Self-Efficacy to Resist Self-Injury and Engage in Alternate Coping Strategies?

Individuals who self-injure can be encouraged to reflect on times when they successfully resisted the urge to self-injure and to consider what was different compared to times they acted on this urge. While these instances are bound to vary, they might involve engaging in self-talk (e.g., *"This feeling will pass, I do not need to self-injure"*), calling a friend, or using another form of coping (e.g., going for a run, taking a hot bath, listening to music). If the factors that reduce the likelihood of acting on urges to self-injure can be identified, these may form the basis of a safety plan an individual can use when the urge to self-injure arises. Importantly, individuals wishing to reduce or stop self-injury should be rewarded for their efforts to resist the urge, even if they still engage in self-injury from time to time. Over time, repeated efforts to resist the urge to self-injure, and rewarding of these, can foster positive self-talk and belief in the ability to resist further urges to self-injure (e.g., *"I have resisted this urge before, I can do it again now"*).

Simultaneously, individuals can be rewarded for attempting alternative coping strategies. Finding alternative strategies that serve the same function as self-injury will take time, effort, and repeated practice. Many individuals who wish to stop or reduce their self-injury fear they will not be able to cope in other ways or that other strategies will not be as effective.[16,17] This lack of self-efficacy to engage alternative coping strategies can present a barrier to building resilience and recovery efforts. As such, even attempts to try other techniques to regulate emotion should be praised. They may not work every time, and this should be explicitly recognized, but as an individual becomes more aware of their emotional experiences, and their potential triggers, they may learn to identify the need for emotion regulation early, providing an opportunity to implement new strategies before the emotional experience becomes too intense. For example, someone who notices they are feeling on edge may opt to go for a run, which will have the effect of reducing their arousal level. This reduction in arousal, or the time to think about what is making them edgy and problem-solve, may be enough to prevent or reduce an urge to self-injure.[18,19] With repeated effort, the belief in the ability to use alternative strategies will increase.

IDENTIFYING STRENGTHS

A key tenet of our recovery framework is that it moves away from a deficit-based model to highlight strengths that can be harnessed as assets in the recovery process. Identifying and using these strengths is key to developing the resilience that allows people to face life's challenges. These strengths could be resources an individual has at their disposal (e.g., support network, coping strategies), beliefs and values (e.g., self-worth, sense of meaning and purpose), or character strengths that pervade thoughts, feelings, and behaviors (e.g., wisdom, courage).[20] Rather than focus on individual deficits, the field of positive psychology focuses on individual differences in positive traits and attributes. In developing a system of classifying these character traits, Peterson and Seligman[21] identified 24 pervasive strengths reflecting six core virtues: (1) Wisdom and knowledge, (2) Courage, (3) Humanity, (4) Justice, (5) Temperance, and (6) Transcendence. These character strengths have been associated with well-being among adolescents[22] and adults,[20,23] and protect against both depression and suicidal thoughts and behaviors.[24] A common exercise is to ask individuals to rank the strengths in order of the degree to which they believe they possess them, using the Values in Action Inventory of Strengths (Table 12.3). This offers people a wide range of areas in which they can demonstrate strengths and emphasizes they do not need to be "perfect" in all areas.

Table 12.3. CHARACTER STRENGTHS CAN BE RANKED IN TERMS OF THE DEGREE
TO WHICH AN INDIVIDUAL POSSESSES THAT STRENGTH.

Core Virtues	Character Strengths	Ranking of Prevalence (1–24)[a]
Wisdom and knowledge	1. Creativity	
	2. Curiosity	
	3. Judgment	
	4. Love of learning	
	5. Perspective	
Courage	6. Bravery	
	7. Honesty	
	8. Perseverance	
	9. Zest	
Humanity	10. Kindness	
	11. Love	
	12. Social intelligence	
Justice	13. Fairness	
	14. Leadership	
	15. Teamwork	
Temperance	16. Forgiveness	
	17. Humility	
	18. Prudence	
	19. Self-regulation	
Transcendence	20. Appreciation of beauty	
	21. Gratitude	
	22. Hope	
	23. Humor	
	24. Spirituality	

[a]Ranking of prevalence could be with regard to specific situations or periods of time.
A rank of 24 indicates the strength is more prevalent

Sometimes it is difficult for people to identify their strengths, particularly if they have a tendency to be self-critical, which is often the case with individuals who self-injure.[25] Further, in situations of heightened distress, working memory capacity can be limited by ongoing rumination about the distressing situation, limiting the ability to generate alternative solutions or refocus on strengths rather than the current emotion. It may therefore be helpful for individuals who self-injure (perhaps together with a clinician, family member, or friend) to identify strengths and prepare a list that can be kept on hand (e.g., on their phone/tablet, in in a journal, on a sheet of paper in a wallet). In times of heightened distress, an individual then has this list with them to refer to, negating the need to identify strengths when cognitive load is already high.

This strengths-based approach also lends itself to targeted interventions. Given the largely deficit-based field of literature, it is perhaps not surprising that there is not a large body of work exploring how character strengths relate to self-injury. Recent work has suggested that gratitude and hope, in particular, are associated with self-injury.[26] Gratitude journals, in which individuals write things they are grateful for each day, are associated with reductions in anxiety, depression, and distress.[27,28] Similarly, exercises such as writing a letter of gratitude to someone, writing down three good things in life, and using character strengths in a new way are associated with increased happiness and reduced depression.[29] Journal and diary interventions designed to reduce self-criticism and enhance self-worth demonstrate reductions in self-injury, although these effects are not maintained long-term.[30]

In addition to identifying and using character strengths, individuals can actively engage with their environment, to find meaning in what they do, and recognize accomplishments across a range of areas. Seligman's PERMA model[31] identifies five components that promote well-being, namely:

- Positive Emotion: Encouraging individuals to savor times they feel happy, hopeful, love, and interest in things
- Engagement: Becoming completely absorbed in activities and living in the moment
- Relationships: Connecting with other people
- Meaning: Finding a purpose in life or getting involved in a cause or organization
- Accomplishments: Setting goals and reflecting on past successes

Individuals can identify the extent to which they have strengths in each of these areas, and actively take steps to engage with others, and reward themselves for achieving goals. These do not need to be big goals. Rather, we recommend SMART goals as outlined below:

Specific (clearly defining what the desired outcome is)
Measurable (to ensure one can tell when the goal has been achieved)
Achievable (goals need to be realistic and attainable)
Relevant (goals should align with interests and values)
Time bound (set a target date by which the goal will be achieved)

Again, it is important to start small and thus with goals that are manageable. For example, setting a goal to get fit is not specific or time-bound and is less likely to result in action to achieve this goal. Likewise, setting a goal to run a marathon may not be achievable in the short term. Instead, someone could set a goal to go for a walk twice a week. These goals need to be tailored to the individual, considering their physical and mental capacities at the time (e.g., if they have depression), and ensure they do not set someone up for failure. Meeting goals should be rewarded, and goals can be reviewed and adapted as circumstances change. Setting, and meeting, goals can give individuals a sense of achievement, building and reinforcing existing strengths and developing new ones.

FINDING ALTERNATIVES TO SELF-INJURY

Finding alternatives to self-injury is not an easy or quick process. It will take time, and effort, and will not always be successful. Our model of self-injury recovery makes this explicit and recognizes that recovery is not a linear process. Self-injury provides a quick and effective (at least in the short term) means of regulating emotion. As such, finding alternatives that serve the same function in the same time frame can be challenging. There are three ways to think about alternatives to self-injury: (1) Reducing the urge to self-injure, (2) Reappraising the urge to self-injure, and (3) Developing alternative coping strategies.

Reducing the Urge to Self-Injure

Incorporating self-care into daily routines is one way to maintain a healthy life-style and promote well-being. By doing so, individuals may find they have more inner resources available to cope with stressful situations, emotional turmoil, or adversity. Self-care includes eating a healthy diet, getting sufficient sleep, regularly exercising, and taking time to engage in enjoyable activities. Poor sleep quality, nightmares, and insomnia have all been associated with self-injury, particularly among adolescents.[32-34] An early case study highlighted the benefit of exercise in reducing self-injury; the patient reported a reduced frequency of self-injury when regularly exercising, which increased again when she ceased exercising.[19] Among adolescents and young adults, physical activity is associated with less frequent self-injury, and moderates the relation between depression and self-injury.[18] Regular exercise has long been considered protective against depression,[35] and reducing depressive symptoms is likely to reduce the urge to self-injure.

One important skill that can help minimize urges to self-injure is emotional awareness. There is some research to suggest that changes in negative affect can be detected hours before an individual self-injures, and up to 7 hours before they report an urge to self-injure.[36] This provides a critical window of opportunity; if individuals can learn to recognize this increase in negative affect they can implement alternative strategies to downregulate emotion, before the urge to self-injure is felt. One way to do this is to check in with emotions on at least a daily basis. Ask: *"What am I feeling?" Why do I feel that way?" What do I need to change how I am feeling?"* Over time an individual can learn to be more in touch with their emotions and recognize when active emotion regulation is needed.

Some people find that regularly journaling, getting their thoughts and emotions onto the page, can be cathartic, and help them recognize what they are feeling, why they are feeling it, and what they need to change how they are feeling. While most individuals who self-injure will not require intensive treatment, the skills training at the core of dialectical behavior therapy may have benefits for everyone.[37] This skills training focuses on enhancing capability in mindfulness, distress tolerance, interpersonal effectiveness, and emotion regulation. Development of these skills will provide individuals with more preventative strategies in their toolkit, allowing them to build resilience in responding to emotional experiences, and reducing urges to self-injure.

Reappraising the Urge to Self-Injure

As noted above, ongoing thoughts and urges to self-injure are a normal part of the recovery process. Resisting these thoughts and urges can be challenging, but there are strategies people can put in place to help reduce self-injury. These include reappraising or reframing the thoughts, in much the same way we suggest reframing instances of self-injury. Normalizing such thoughts and recognizing that thoughts do not necessarily lead to action is important (e.g., *"Having thoughts of self-injury is perfectly normal, but I do not need to act on them"*). Recognizing that thoughts will come and go is also important. If the urge to self-injure arises an individual may be able to wait 15 minutes before acting on this urge. During this 15 minutes they may find their arousal subsides, or they become distracted and the urge diminished, even if not reduced entirely.

Relatedly, urge surfing is a technique commonly used in the field of substance dependence.[2] This involves noticing an urge, and then rather than trying to fight it, noticing the associated feelings and using meditation techniques to "ride" the urge, like riding a wave as it rises and wanes as it comes into shore. A large body of work demonstrates that suppressing thoughts or urges often increases distress and focuses more attention on the behavior we are trying to avoid.[38-39] By accepting the urge, and accepting it without judgment, the urge is given less importance and eventually diminishes. With practice, urge surfing becomes easier and contributes to a sense of self-efficacy and resilience.

Developing Alternative Coping Strategies

Ultimately, finding alternatives to self-injury requires development of a coping repertoire with a range of strategies that can be used in different situations when individuals are feeling overwhelmed. Different strategies are going to work for different people, and different strategies are more or less appropriate in different contexts. Almost any coping strategy that does not cause harm to oneself or others is worth a try at least once. As noted above, development of emotional awareness and early detection of distress provides a window of opportunity for individuals to implement another coping strategy, potentially reducing the urge to self-injure.

Active problem-solving may be one technique that individuals can use to identify the source of distress and work to address the underlying issue rather than reeling in the emotional consequences. The steps in problem-solving include:

1. **Identify the problem:** be as specific and concrete as possible.
2. **Generate as many solutions as possible:** these do not need to be realistic or achievable; the idea is simply to brainstorm any options that might help address the problem,

3. **Select a solution:** at this point it does help if the solution is achievable!
4. **Implement and evaluate the solution:** did it work to address the problem? Why or why not? What could be done next time the situation arises?

Choosing alternative coping strategies when particularly overwhelmed, down, or irritated can be more challenging. Although avoidant coping strategies are typically associated with less favorable outcomes,[40] it may be that distraction from the situation, thoughts, and/or emotion may be beneficial in the context of self-injury. This might mean going to the movies, cleaning the house, or calling a friend. Regardless of the strategy chosen or the approach employed, practicing new coping skills takes considerable time and conscious effort.

Another approach may be to develop a Safety or Support Plan. These plans can be completed alone, or in conjunction with others (family, friend, therapist) and are considered gold standard practice is working with individuals who express suicidal thoughts.[41] Although self-injury is not about suicide, the fundamental principles still apply. A template for a support plan is provided in Chapter 2. The idea is to complete this plan in a calm and quiet environment, when feeling relaxed. Then, when a person has an urge to self-injure they may access this plan rather than having to come up with alternatives on the spot. Importantly, support plans can be iterative, such that they are matched to the level of intensity of the emotion being experienced. For example, someone who ranks their distress as 10/10 is not going to be calmed by quietly sitting and reading a book. They may need to pour cold water over their head or take a cold shower to shock the body into reducing their physiological arousal. This may result in their distress now being ranked at 8/10. At this point, they may decide that talking to a friend would be helpful; this may reduce distress to 6/10. Once distress is incrementally lower, the alternative activities can also be lowered in intensity.

UNDERLYING ADVERSITIES

Although not always associated with mental illness, self-injury is typically associated with psychological distress and/or difficulties in regulating emotion and coping. As such, recovery efforts will likely include efforts to improve emotion regulation and coping. In cases where self-injury is associated with underlying psychological concerns then treatment may be needed to address these concerns. Here treatment may focus on the primary issues (e.g., anxiety, depression, trauma) rather than the self-injury per se. As such, we do not recommend any individual therapeutic approach but suggest individuals seek a therapist and an approach that works for them. If self-injury is being used to cope with these underlying concerns, then it is likely self-injury will reduce as the primary mental health needs are addressed.

SCARRING

Not all individuals with a history of self-injury will have visible scarring, and some may have scars that are visible to themselves but not to others. We argue that for individuals who do have scarring, part of the self-injury recovery process involves understanding their relationship with and the meaning attributed to these visible signs of self-injury.[42-43] For some individuals self-injury scars are associated with shame, disgust, and lack of self-acceptance. For others, scars are seen as a sign of resilience, or a reminder that they have survived tough times. Further, individuals with self-injury scars can have very mixed views about their scars (e.g., a love/hate relationship).[44,45]

These mixed views are probably not surprising considering the significant stigma associated with self-injury and with self-injury scars specifically. In experimental work, individuals demonstrate stronger negative reactions to self-injury scars than to socially accepted forms of body modification (e.g., tattoos), or scars incurred through accident.[46] The self-reported psychosocial impact of self-injury is associated with the extent of scarring,[44] and concealment of scars is associated with more negative scar cognitions, anxiety, and depression.[47]

The decision to no longer conceal visible scars can be a significant one for an individual with lived experience of self-injury. Stigma is more likely associated with behaviors that are considered under the individuals' control, and those viewed as visually unpleasant. For this reason, self-injury may attract more stigma than other behaviors that are more easily hidden.[48] Self-compassion and self-acceptance of scars then is critical to countering public stigma and allowing an individual the freedom to be themselves.

Acceptance and commitment therapy,[49] which focuses on reducing shame and fostering self-acceptance, seems particularly pertinent to addressing any experiences of shame associated with self-injury scars. As with many other factors outlined in this chapter, a cognitive reframing of what scars mean can be helpful in guiding an individual toward accepting their scars. Rather than focusing on reminders of past negative experiences, scars can be reframed as a sign of resilience for making it through those experiences. This reframing may also be a useful tool to use if a person does experience stigma as a result of visible self-injury scars.

DISCLOSURE

Alongside acceptance of scarring, self-injury recovery necessitates consideration of disclosure of lived experience of self-injury. Disclosure may be voluntary or involuntary, or be made by a third party. While involuntary disclosures (e.g., other people noticing scars) can be difficult to control, there are many factors to consider in the decision to voluntarily disclose a history of self-injury, or ongoing self-injury (see Table 12.4). Theoretical models of disclosure in the broader health

Table 12.4. FACTORS TO CONSIDER IN THE DECISION TO DISCLOSE SELF-INJURY.

Motivations	Self-Injury Characteristics	Interpersonal Factors	Self-Efficacy	Psychological Outcomes	Social Outcomes	Setting the Scene
• Why do I want to disclose self-injury?	• Do I have self-injury scars that are visible to others?	• Is it relevant to the other person?	• Do I have the strength to disclose self-injury?	• How do I expect to feel after I disclose my self-injury?	• How will disclosure impact this relationship?	• Where and when will I disclose my self-injury?
• What do I hope will happen when I disclose?	• Do I continue to self-injure?	• Do they need to know?	• What words will I use to tell the other person?	• What are the good outcomes that could occur?	• Will disclosure have any impact on other areas of my life (e.g., work)?	• Choose a quiet & comfortable location where you will have plenty of time and not be interrupted.
• What do I actually want to communicate?	• Would I consider myself "recovered"?	• How well do I know this person?		• What are the less favorable outcomes that could occur?		
	• Are there underlying psychological concerns or thoughts of suicide that accompany my self-injury?	• How close is the relationship?		• What will I do if there is a poor outcome?		
		• What do I expect the other person to do or say in response to disclosure?		• How will this impact the way I view my self-injury story?		

field (e.g., disclosure of a cancer diagnosis) outline a number of factors that feed into the decision to voluntarily disclose the information.

In the disclosure decision-making model, Greene[50] first considers the information to be disclosed. This includes considering the extent to which the information is stigmatized, the symptoms and prognosis, and the relevance of the information to others. These factors are interrelated and will be more or less relevant depending on the information to disclose. For example, relevance to others may be important in disclosing a sexually transmitted infection, but may be less relevant to disclosure of self-injury. In the context of self-injury, the concepts of symptoms and prognosis may be thought of as the extent of visible scarring, or potential association with underlying psychological distress, or suicidal thoughts. Greene also highlights the importance of the receiver of the information and the quality of the relationship with this person. A final component in the decision to disclose information is a person's self-efficacy to disclose. If people do not feel they have the ability to disclose the information they are less likely to decide to disclose it.

Extending this thinking, Chaudoir and Fisher[51] proposed a model of disclosure decision-making that included both antecedents and consequences of disclosure. Notably, they focus on antecedent goals—or what a person intends to achieve through disclosure. Like Greene,[50] they recognize the importance of the content of the disclosure and the relationship with the person receiving a disclosure, but extend this to consider the short- and long-term outcomes of disclosure for the individual, their relationship with the person receiving the disclosure, and broader society. Last, they propose that alleviation of inhibition (similar to self-efficacy to disclose), social support, and the potential for shared information to impact social interactions mediate the relations between the disclosure event and its outcomes.

Applied to voluntary disclosure of self-injury, similar factors should be considered. As outlined in Table 12.4, when thinking about disclosing lived experience of self-injury to another person it is important to think about the motives underlying the disclosure. Understanding why one is considering disclosure may drive how the information is disclosed, and what the outcome might be. Thinking about where one is in the recovery process may also be a factor to consider. At the very least this may underlie what information is disclosed and whether there is likely to be ongoing disclosure of self-injury. Importantly, the relationship with the person to receive the disclosure should be considered. This may also factor into considerations of the likely outcome of disclosure.

Individuals should prepare for both positive and less favorable outcomes. Someone may react in a supportive and nonjudgmental manner to a person disclosing self-injury. Alternatively, they may express shock, fear, or disgust. Parents, in particular, can have their own reactions to finding out their child self-injures, reporting anxiety, questioning their parenting, and wondering how they did not know their child was self-injuring.[52,53] Having a plan in place to cope with any negative reactions that may arise from disclosure may be helpful. This might mean planning to call a friend, go for a walk, or make time to talk to the disclosure recipient at a later date when they have had time to process this new information.

Individuals could also consider the positive outcomes; individuals have told us that although they anticipate negative reactions to disclosure they are often surprised at the supportive response they receive.[54] Concealment of self-injury can involve constant vigilance and censoring on the part of the person with lived experience. Although not a lot of empirical work has explored positive impacts of disclosure beyond receiving support or sharing their experiences, it is plausible that disclosure allows an individual with lived experience to feel more authentic in their interactions with others, and in doing so begin to foster self-acceptance.

SELF-ACCEPTANCE

While individuals may fear they will not be accepted by others if their self-injury is known, it may be more important to foster self-acceptance than rely on acceptance from others. Self-acceptance involves unconditionally accepting oneself—warts and all—and for someone with lived experience of self-injury this will also include acceptance of this experience. There is no judgment of the self as "good" or "bad," but simply accepting oneself for who they are. It's easy to be critical of the things we do not like about ourselves. So self-acceptance might start by taking a look at strengths (see above) and values. Individuals might also consider things they cannot control, and learn to minimize focus on these. Ruminating on things that cannot be changed only causes distress. Instead, people can control how they feel and respond to situations that are out of their control. Some people find it helpful to list things they do not like about themselves, but to reframe how they think about them. For example, rather than saying "I hate the way I look, I've put on so much weight," this could be reframed as: "Everybody is different and has a unique look. I've always loved running; maybe I can take that up again." A strengths focus that is encouraging and coupled with a goal is more likely to foster change than self-criticism.

A related idea is self-compassion. Individuals often find it easy to feel compassion for others, but are reluctant to show compassion to themselves. According to Kristen Neff[55] there are three elements of self-compassion: (1) Self-kindness, (2) Common humanity, and (3) Mindfulness. Being kind to oneself when things are not going well is seen as the compassionate alternative to self-judgment and self-criticism. A recognition that suffering is part of the human condition means accepting our imperfections and realizing that no one is perfect. Mindfulness allows people to take a more balanced and nonjudgmental approach to emotions, rather than trying to avoid or ignore them.

There are several ways in which individuals can practice self-compassion. Kristen Neff's website (self-compassion.org) provides a number of self-compassion exercises. These include:

1. **How would you treat a friend?**—thinking about how you would respond to a friend who is going through a tough time and thinking about how you could respond to yourself in the same way

2. **Self-compassion break**—taking 3 minutes to be mindful of suffering, recognize that suffering is part of life, and seeking to be kind to yourself
3. **Exploring self-compassion through writing**—including writing a letter to yourself from the perspective of a loving imaginary friend
4. **Supportive touch**—this could involve taking some deep breathes and placing a hand over the heart to notice the natural rise and fall of the chest
5. **Changing your critical self-talk**—reframing your critical inner voice to be more kind and positive
6. **Self-compassion journal**—keeping a daily diary focused on mindfulness, common humanity, and self-kindness
7. **Identify what we really want**—rather than using self-criticism as a motivator, reframe this criticism into a voice that is encouraging and supportive
8. **Taking care of the caregiver**—giving yourself permission to care for yourself as well as for others

These exercises might seem a little strange and uncomfortable at first for some individuals; this is understandable and ought to be normalized. But there is a growing body of research to show that self-compassion is related to psychological well-being.[56] Interventions that adopt a self-compassion framework have also demonstrated improvements in rumination, depression, eating behaviors, stress, criticism, and anxiety.[57] Self-compassion exercises may not be everyone's cup of tea—but they are worth trying as part of an ongoing repertoire of skills to target self-critical thought. Taking our person-centered approach, self-compassion will be a better fit for some than others, and as with other elements of the framework, individuals will need to find approaches that work best for them.

CONCLUSION

As outlined in Chapter 11, self-injury recovery is not a simple or linear process. What is important to bear in mind is that recovery goes well beyond simply ceasing to self-injure. The recovery process will be different for each person. Some may learn to accept scarring before fully believing they can resist urges to self-injure. Some may be able to identify their strengths before addressing underlying psychological concerns. Some may disclose their self-injury before accepting that thoughts of self-injury may be ongoing. Some may never disclose their self-injury to others, but learn self-acceptance and practice self-compassion. It is our hope that the strategies outlined in this chapter will be helpful to individuals, and those who care for them, in thinking about self-injury recovery, and in taking concrete steps to build resilience.

Supporting People With Lived Experience

As mentioned in Chapter 4, the stigmatization of self-injury remains ubiquitous and significant. Such stigma makes it difficult for people to reach out about their experience, even when they may want support. Further, many people who do not have lived experience, but who are concerned about someone who does, want to lend support but are uncertain about how to navigate this; they do not know what to say or how to offer support. We therefore focus this chapter on the application of a person-centered approach when discussing self-injury that can be used during interactions with individuals who have lived experience. Drawing on these recommendations can help foster more appropriate discussions about self-injury and, thus, leave individuals with lived experience feeling more understood and validated. After presenting this approach, we touch on other ways that people can support individuals who have lived experience of self-injury; this includes addressing overshadowed concerns that have salience to people with lived experience.

CONVERSATIONS ABOUT SELF-INJURY: APPLYING A PERSON-CENTERED APPROACH

When applying a person-centered approach to support individuals who engage in self-injury it is important to keep in mind that they are experts in their *own* lived experience.[1,2] Although this may appear obvious on the surface, having this in one's awareness helps to avoid the possible influence of preconceived notions about why a person self-injures, what self-injury may mean to that person, or how that individual ought to navigate *their* experience. This includes avoiding well-intentioned attempts to problem-solve a person's difficulties (e.g., jumping in to offer advice about how someone can stop self-injury). Such approaches may come across as though one is not listening. This may, in turn, shut down future conversations. Hence, it is vital that attention be mindfully paid to the person's expressed needs, concerns, and experiences and that this is done without judgment. Findings from our research have indicated that many individuals will be worried about being judged for having self-injured or that their engagement in the behavior will take precedence in terms of how they are viewed.[1,3,4] Ultimately, there is more to a person's story than self-injury.[1,3–5] Thus, each individual ought to be viewed holistically—as a full person.[1] With this in mind, we now turn to recommended approaches for the application of a person-centered approach to discuss self-injury. The key components of this approach are summarized in Figure 13.1.

First and foremost, it is essential that any discussion about self-injury occur without judgment.[1,6–9] Hence, one should endeavor to communicate empathy and a corresponding desire to understand a person's experience.[1] Critical to this is communicating genuine interest in understanding another person's experience, which can be accomplished by using a *respectful curiosity* that situates the individual as an expert in their own experience (see Chapters 2 and 10).[1,6–9] Accordingly, one would seek to learn about and understand a person's experience without judgment. To facilitate this, one can use questions that convey a genuine interest in understanding aspects of another's experience (e.g., *Could you help me understand how self-injury works for you? I'd like to try and understand what makes it hard for you to talk about self-injury. Could you help me understand what makes it difficult for you?*). By using this approach, people with lived experience are afforded space to articulate their own experience and concerns without assumption, expectation, or judgment. In concert with this, it can be helpful to explicitly acknowledge that conversations about self-injury can be difficult.[1] Doing so works to validate the individual and their experience, while allaying worry about how people may react.

Although discussions about self-injury will clearly involve at least some attention to a person's experience with the behavior, it is recommended this should

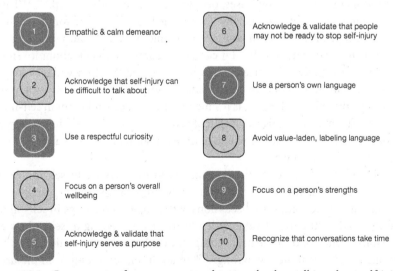

Figure 13.1. Components of a person-centered approach when talking about self-injury.

not be the sole focus.[1] Rather, attention should also be placed on a person's overall well-being. Too much emphasis on self-injury can be counterproductive for a few reasons. First, if the conversation becomes too detailed, it can be triggering and upsetting for some people (e.g., excessive focus on self-injury methods or moments in which self-injury was enacted). Second, too much attention on self-injury can leave a person feeling as though any other concerns or difficulties pertinent to their experience are not as important or that there is no space for them to be raised. To avoid this, it can be helpful to overtly communicate concern for a person's overall well-being, along with questions about their experience[1] (e.g., *I'm concerned about how you're doing overall and want to make sure you're okay*).

As conversations unfold, and more about one's experience with self-injury is shared, several other components of a person-centered approach are likely to be relevant. Consistent with expressing recognition that discussions about self-injury can be difficult, it is also important to validate that self-injury serves a purpose (or several purposes) for people who self-injure.[3] Often, individuals with lived experience believe that other people will not be able to understand why they self-injure or that upon knowing more about their experience, judgment will ensue.[1,3] Validating someone's reasons for self-injury can thus go a long way in mollifying these concerns.[1] In keeping with the uniqueness of each person's experience, including the reason(s) for their self-injury, people will inevitably use different words when describing their experiences with self-injury—including the term(s) used to refer to the behavior itself. Using and reflecting back a person's exact framings during a conversation helps to validate their experience;[1,6-8] doing so also circumvents any unintended "correcting" of a their experience (e.g., using a term that does not align with a person's experience).

Although it is absolutely possible for people to recover and find meaning from their experience of self-injury and any related adversities, stopping self-injury can be quite difficult.[5,10,11] In many cases, people will not be ready to stop.[5,10-13] This is certainly understandable—especially if someone has self-injured for an extended time. Indeed, prior difficulty in stopping or being unready to stop self-injury altogether may exacerbate how hard it can be for someone to talk about it.[1] In this regard, people with lived experience may be concerned that they will be asked (or at times, told) to stop. Acknowledging that a person may not be ready to stop self-injuring can therefore be helpful as it validates the difficulty inherent in self-injury cessation.[1] Furthermore, this can implicitly communicate that self-injury serves a purpose and that, as a result, it will take time for someone to find alternatives to take the place of self-injury.

As discussed in Chapter 5, the language used in reference to self-injury and people with lived experience is critical for numerous reasons. This is perhaps especially relevant in the context of discussions with people who engage in self-injury.[1] Of note, avoiding the use of value-laden terms (e.g., referring to self-injury as a maladaptive behavior or unhelpful coping strategy) can inadvertently convey that what one is doing is somehow wrong.[14-16] In addition, refraining from the use of terms that position a person *as* a behavior (e.g., referring to people as self-injurers or cutters) is similarly crucial. These types of referents are reductionistic and they can worsen stigma, making people feel like less of a person.[15-17]

Beyond the above considerations, attention to people's strengths should be woven into all conversations about self-injury.[1] There are a few reasons for this. First, it is not uncommon for people with lived experience to have higher levels of self-criticism.[18] Understandably, this would make it more difficult for people to identify and acknowledge their own strengths. Drawing attention to a person's individual strengths can thus go a long way in countering negative views of oneself.[1] Second, as noted earlier in our book, much of the discourse regarding self-injury is deficit-based. Thus, it is incumbent on everyone to challenge these unhelpful framings, as they may dissuade recovery efforts and leave people feeling further misunderstood and stigmatized. A strengths-based focus in conversations about self-injury represents one potential antidote to these unhelpful framings. Third, we know that a person's recovery journey is nonlinear and will thus wax and wane over time. Setbacks are indeed a part of the process for most people.[2,10,11] Accordingly, intentional focus on people's strengths—including small frontward steps (e.g., when people open-up about difficult experiences, when they mention times during which they had an urge to self-injure but did not hurt themselves)— can play a key role in sustaining a person's recovery efforts and efficacy. In clinical contexts, attention to these kinds of strengths (and cheerleading them) can likewise work to maintain people's engagement in the therapeutic process.

Broaching the Topic and Ongoing Conversations

Many of the components of the person-centered approach described above have relevance when a discussion about self-injury has been initiated (e.g., validating that self-injury serves a purpose). However, they can also be applied when one has concern about another's self-injury but is unsure how to broach the topic. As discussed before, it is not uncommon for people with lived experience to express reluctance about sharing their experience (even if they may want to).[3] In such cases, it may be up to someone else to raise the topic—a prospect that is clearly easier said than done. To facilitate this, it may be first helpful to reflect on any potential biases or preconceived notions that one may have about self-injury (e.g., thinking about what one knows about it, identifying any beliefs one might have about why people self-injure). It is also recommended that one read about self-injury from reputable sources to ensure that they develop a working foundation of knowledge about what self-injury is (and is not), why someone might self-injure, and so forth. From here, it is important to bear in mind that conversations about self-injury should occur when there is time to actively listen to a person's experience. These conversations should never be rushed (e.g., it would not be advised for someone to begin a conversation when driving that person to work or school).

When starting any dialogue, many of the aforementioned principles of a person-centered approach can be drawn on (e.g., conveying a respectful curiosity).[1] Framing initial questions in this regard can therefore be helpful. For example, rather than asking a direct question (e.g., *Do you self-injure? Are you cutting yourself?*), it is recommended that the question be put into a greater context (e.g., in recognition of a person's recent changes in mood, indicators that someone might be self-injuring); by doing so, concern about a person's overall well-being should be highlighted. For example, one might ask *"I've noticed that you've been more withdrawn and have noticed cuts on your arm and I'm concerned about how you're doing. I know that some people may turn to self-injury when having difficulty coping and am wondering if this is what is going on for you?"* Asking questions like this, while using a nonjudgmental tone, allows someone to open up dialogue about self-injury in a way that is much less likely to come across as an interrogation and instead as a genuine attempt to understand another's experience while also expressing concern for that person. Moreover, putting the initial question into context (e.g., grounding a question in what one has noticed recently) minimizes the potential that a question be construed as though a person is being blamed for having self-injured.

Along with the above, it should be recognized that much like someone may not be ready to stop self-injury, a person may also not be prepared to talk about it. It may (and often does) take time to open up about one's experiences with self-injury. Because of this, it can be helpful to convey to someone with lived experience that it is okay if they are not ready to talk. Likewise, it should also be communicated that one will be available to talk when that person is ready (perhaps, even reiterating this so it is not forgotten and that future opportunities to talk will be available). It is important to bear in mind that conversations about self-injury will often occur over multiple time points versus a single sitting. In Box 13.1, we present example questions that readers may find useful when applying a person-centered approach during interactions about self-injury.

Box 13.1.

EXAMPLE QUESTIONS FOR A PERSON-CENTERED APPROACH WHEN TALKING ABOUT SELF-INJURY.

Acknowledge and validate that self-injury is difficult to talk about

- I recognize that talking about self-injury can be really hard for people. However, I would like to understand more and learn about your experience.
- I can tell this is tough for you to talk about and appreciate that you're willing to talk to me about this.
- I appreciate that self-injury is difficult to talk about and want you to know that I'm here for you and here to listen when you're ready.

Use a respectful curiosity when asking questions

- I've noticed that you are much more withdrawn lately. It also seems like you're having a hard time coping. I know that when this happens some people may hurt themselves. I'm curious, is this happening for you?
- I care about you and am concerned about how you're doing. I've noticed that you aren't talking as much with me. I have also seen some cuts on your arm and am wondering if you are hurting yourself?
- I'd like to better understand your experience. Can you help me understand how self-injury works for you?
- It seems like this is hard to talk about. Can you help me understand what makes it hard for you to talk about self-injury with me?
- I've heard that when people are struggling to cope, they may use self-injury. I'm wondering if this is going on for you?

Acknowledge and validate that self-injury serves a purpose

- Based on what you've said it seems that self-injury allows you to feel a bit better when you get really upset and overwhelmed.
- I can appreciate why you feel you have to cut yourself when you get so upset. It sounds like it's really hard to cope sometimes.

Acknowledge and validate that a person may not be ready to stop self-injury

- It sounds like there's a lot going on and that it really feels overwhelming at times. I can see how this would make it hard to stop self-injury.
- It's not uncommon for people to say that they are unsure about stopping self-injury. I think it makes sense that you'd be going back and forth about this.
- Given what you've said about having no other way to cope, I can understand that you'd feel as though you are not quite ready to stop self-harming.

Use a person's language

- If a person specifically mentions "cutting" or another term such as "my self-harm" use that term when asking questions (e.g., Can you help me understand a bit about what cutting/your self-harm does for you?)

Refrain from using value-laden, labeling language

- The following referents should be avoided: calling self-injury a maladaptive, unhealthy, or dysfunctional behavior or coping strategy; referring to people as cutters, self-injurers, self-harmers

Focus on people's strengths

- Draw attention to prior instances when someone had an urge, but it was not acted on (this is especially important when someone has difficulty identifying these occurrences)
- Highlight when people open-up about their experience or to try new coping strategies, acknowledging the strength/courage/effort to do so

SUPPORTING INDIVIDUALS WITH LIVED EXPERIENCE: OTHER CONSIDERATIONS

Professional Help

At different junctures—including initial and ongoing discussions—the topic of professional help-seeking may emerge. In some cases, the person offering support may want to recommend that someone seek professional help; in other cases, someone might express their views about seeking professional help when opening up about their self-injury (e.g., trepidation about talking to a mental health professional, uncertainty about how to seek help, a strong desire to talk to a professional). Given this, it can be helpful to become familiar with some of the local resources and professional supports that are available in one's area. By doing so, if the aspect of professional help-seeking is raised, a person with lived experience can be directed to relevant points of contact.

Importantly, professional help should not be pushed or discussed in a way that comes across as a mandate, especially if a person with lived experience is concerned about talking to a professional. If this is forced, it may devolve the conversation and drive someone away from future dialogue about self-injury. People should be able to make their own choice about obtaining professional help and seeking treatment. Accordingly, it would be important to validate concerns that people might have about speaking with a professional and to normalize that this is common and understandable (especially if someone has had an unhelpful or adverse clinical experience). It would also be important to acknowledge that although some people have reservations about seeking professional help, many people find it beneficial. In tandem with this, it can be useful to communicate that it can take time to find a "good fit" when it comes to talking to and working with a helping professional. If individuals know that it may take time to find the right person for them to work with, they may be less dissuaded in the event an initial encounter with a professional does not unfold as anticipated.

Although many people can and do benefit from seeking professional help for self-injury and any underlying or associated difficulties, not everyone will be ready for this. Should this be the case, it can be helpful to also be aware of reputable online resources that can be shared with someone with lived experience. These can not only provide helpful information about self-injury but also offer ways to cope with urges and triggers. Often, online information about self-injury also addresses treatment-seeking; this may prove useful when addressing someone's concerns or uncertainty about help-seeking. With this in mind, we have outlined several reputable resources that may offer utility in these instances in Box 13.2.

Box 13.2

Self-Injury Outreach and Support (SiOS)
www.sioutreach.org

The SiOS website offers a range of research-informed resources geared toward individuals with lived experience of self-injury, including a set of coping guides (e.g., coping with urges, coping day-to-day) as well as recovery stories and words of inspiration from other people who have self-injured. SiOS also has information and guides for other stakeholders, namely: families, friends, romantic partners, schools, and health and mental professionals.

Cornell Research Program on Self-Injury and Recovery
www.selfinjury.bctr.cornell.edu

The Cornell Research Program on Self-injury and Recovery houses a large set of research-informed resources and guides about self-injury (e.g., coping strategies, information about disclosure, information about recovery and seeking treatment). In addition, this site provides an array of resources and guides for various stakeholders, including but not limited to families, schools, and professionals.

SAFE Alternatives
www.selfinjury.com

Based in the United States, SAFE Alternatives is a treatment approach for self-injury. In addition to offering information about this form of treatment, their website offers content for people who self-injure and those who support them (e.g., families, health professionals).

Shedding Light on Self-Injury
www.self-injury.org.au

This site is based in Australia and provides research-informed information for health professionals who work with individuals who self-injure, in addition to general resources for people to learn more information about self-injury.

The Mighty's Guide to Understanding Self-Harm
https://themighty.com/topic/self-harm/what-is-self-harm

The Mighty is a large online community that brings together people who live with a range of physical and mental health difficulties and illnesses. On this specific part of their website, they have consolidated information from research and interviews with leading experts in the field of self-injury. This includes recovery-oriented material for individuals with lived experience of self-injury alongside content for concerned loved ones.

Note: This box mirrors Table 7.1 as the websites listed are relevant to readers of both chapters.

Scarring

In the context of supporting someone with lived experience of self-injury, some individuals may express concerns about having scars from self-injury. Indeed, scarring from self-injury has been identified as a significant concern for many people.[19-23] For example, someone may be worried about how other people will react if their scars are noticed in a public or work setting. In other instances, people may have experienced times when someone did notice (or seemed to) and found that experience very difficult. And in other cases, someone may have difficulty coming to terms with their scars and feel shame or embarrassment about them. In each of these scenarios, drawing on elements of a person-centered approach (e.g., a nonjudgmental approach, conveying empathy) can help to validate that person's concerns and demonstrate that while many people have reservations about others seeing their scars, not everyone will react negatively (e.g., *Based on what you've shared, I can appreciate that you'd be worried about how people might react to your scars. That sounds difficult and I'd like to understand a bit more of what that's like for you*). From here, dialogue about a person's scar-related concerns can be facilitated using a respectful curiosity (e.g., *You mentioned that you're worried about having scars from self-injury. Can you help me understand what makes you worried about your scars?*).

Related to having scarring, some people may ask for advice about how or whether to conceal their scars. Likewise, they may ponder openly displaying their scars as a part of their recovery experience. As outlined earlier in the book, the decision to hide or make one's scars visible is a deeply personal one. Therefore, it is important to avoid jumping into offering advice (e.g., outright dissuading the showing of one's scars). Much as we discussed earlier for conversations about self-injury, it would also be important to reflect on one's own views to avoid forcing that perspective on someone who has self-injury scarring. For example, a person in a supportive role may believe that showing scars in public is a bad decision. If this comes across as an undertone of any scar-related conversations, it may inadvertently communicate that having scars is somehow bad or wrong and that they must be concealed. If this is implied, it may unintentionally worsen people's feelings of shame or self-stigma. Accordingly, it would be important to instead validate that the choice to hide or show one's scars represents an important but ultimately personal decision; thus, it would be important to encourage that individual to contemplate and weigh the positive (e.g., feeling empowered) and negative (e.g., people asking inappropriate questions, people staring and making someone feel uneasy) consequences of that decision. In the case of the latter, it would also be important for the individual to consider how they might cope with and manage instances in which there is a negative reaction to one's scars (e.g., being able to reach out to a friend, using an established coping strategy). Collectively, by drawing on elements of a person-centered approach during these conversations, individuals with lived experience of self-injury will likely feel more validated and will thus be better positioned to take the time needed to make an informed decision that best suits them. In some cases, this is also a decision that can be made with the support of a professional; thus, when a person is seeking treatment, scarring could be integrated as a part of the therapeutic work undertaken (much like what was discussed in Chapter 12).

Supporting People's Choice About Disclosure

Understandably, individuals with lived experience of self-injury may also debate whether and when to tell others about their self-injury. Much as with scarring, the choice to do this is both significant and personal. Thus, a blanket approach to disclosure should be avoided as there are likely an array of considerations to contemplate (e.g., to whom, what/how much is disclosed, the reason for the disclosure). Indeed, sharing one's experience with self-injury is not a one-shoe-fits-all decision.

To support someone who is debating telling someone else about their self-injury, a person-centered approach may again be useful. Specifically, communicating empathy and being nonjudgmental when having these conversations would be key. Likewise, it would be important to avoid injecting one's own views on a person with lived experience of self-injury and instead seek to understand a person's experience using a respectful curiosity (e.g., *I can appreciate that you want to tell your friend about self-injury. I'd like to understand this a bit more. Can you tell me what is going into your decision?*). As disclosure-related decisions can be difficult, validating any expressed concerns a person is recommended (e.g., *I can tell this is a tough decision. I think that makes sense given what you've told me about your past experience with self-injury*).

Much like what was described for decisions about hiding or showing one's scars, when it comes to disclosure, supporting someone to explore both the positive and potentially negative consequences of the decision would be important. This way, a decision is not made rashly and, instead, the person considers the various ways that the potential disclosure may unfold. Commensurate with this, it would be important that the individual making the decision to share their experience also has a coping plan to implement in the event the disclosure does not transpire as planned. Finally, like with scarring, the choice to share one's experience of self-injury with other people can be supported and addressed in clinical settings. Hence, for people seeking treatment, it can be suggested that another source of support in this decision-making process is to work with their mental health professional.

THE IMPORTANCE OF SELF-CARE

In general, supporting someone who is struggling or facing adversity can be difficult. The same applies when supporting someone who has lived experience of self-injury. This is particularly salient in the context of existing relationships (e.g., between romantic partners or friends). It is therefore critical that people in supportive roles engage in their own self-care. Without this, one's own resources will become depleted and their capacity to offer the support they would like will be limited. To be able to offer support ongoingly, individuals in supportive roles are encouraged to take time for themselves. For example, this could involve continued engagement in hobbies, taking time to exercise, or spending time with important others. It is also important to recognize that in some cases, it may be helpful to seek professionals support for oneself. This may become more relevant when one finds that their own well-being is being negatively impacted and they are having difficulty coping themselves.

CONCLUSION

There are many factors (e.g., stigma) that render self-injury difficult for many people to talk about. Likewise, there are many factors (e.g., uncertainty) that make it difficult for people in supportive roles to know how to appropriately respond or engage in dialogue about self-injury. These barriers notwithstanding, it *is* possible to engage in appropriate communication about self-injury and for people with lived experience to feel heard, supported, and validated in the process—even when there are unique concerns such as scarring and future disclosures. To this end, and given the significance of these conversations, drawing on a person-centered approach is paramount. Not only does the approach outlined in this chapter help to facilitate more effective dialogue, but it also works to mitigate the possibility of people feeling invalidated or misunderstood. Ultimately, adopting this approach during initial and ongoing conversations is essential for optimizing outcomes for *all* individuals involved.

Advocating for a Person-Centered, Strengths-Based Approach

In line with an emerging set of efforts, including calls to the field, there is growing recognition that lived experience 'voices are central to advancing our understanding of self-injury.[1-4] To this end, we have focused this final chapter on providing an overview of similar initiatives in other areas before transitioning to a focus on how this can be achieved in the field of self-injury. This includes acknowledging potential barriers to this kind of work but then offering practical suggestions for the integration of person-centered approaches that emphasize lived experience voices in various domains—including research, clinical practice, and outreach.

BROADER LIVED EXPERIENCE INITIATIVES

Across several fields, including various areas within mental health, there are many examples of established initiatives for the formal inclusion of people with lived experience in empirical, service provision, and outreach contexts. Commensurate with this, the World Health Organization has long advocated for this kind of work to empower people with mental health difficulties who have been historically marginalized based on having a mental health disability. For instance, individuals with lived experience have been involved in a variety of undertakings, such as service delivery and associated decision-making, that not only enhance access to resources and treatment but also yield greater social connectedness, higher self-esteem, and more self-efficacy.

In recognition of the need for lived experience voices, several professional organizations have also dedicated membership sections specifically for individuals with lived experience, such as the Academy for Eating Disorders and American Association for Suicidology, among many others. By virtue of offering these opportunities, people can meet, liaise, and work with other members of major organizations and thus work to ensure that lived experience voices and concerns are represented in agenda setting and decision-making. In a similar vein, the need for lived experience work has been acknowledged in research contexts. Indeed, many granting agencies are now prioritizing funding for research that not only focuses on lived experience but also formally involves people with lived experience in the research process. For example, the Canadian Institute of Health Research (a major funding agency for health and mental health research) has specific funding to support research that is participatory in nature. Taken together, there is growing acknowledgment in many sectors that lived experience voices are integral to advancing a variety of fields.

IMPEDIMENTS TO LIVED EXPERIENCE INITIATIVES IN THE FIELD OF SELF-INJURY

Lived experience work in the field of self-injury is relatively nascent, with only a dearth of formal efforts to date.[1] Yet, increasingly, there is recognition that such efforts may be needed in research, clinical care provision, outreach, and membership in discipline-based organizations and societies.[1-4] To effectively work toward these aims, however, recognition of potential barriers to such work is key.

One notable hurdle to advancing the field of self-injury is stigma.[1] Unsurprisingly, stigma is a well-documented concern for myriad mental health difficulties given its pervasive and profound impact on people with lived experience.[5,6] To address this stigma, numerous initiatives have been enacted to improve mental health literacy and people's understanding of mental illness in society.[7-9] Although most would concur that continued efforts are needed, there has been significant progress in bringing awareness about what mental health difficulties are; public attitudes and perceptions about mental illness are—at least to some degree—changing. For example, mental illness tends to not be viewed as the product of one's failure; likewise, mental health challenges are not readily viewed as something that people should just "get over" and people who struggle with their mental health are not typically seen as weak.

Despite these important advances, stigma remains a major concern in the context of self-injury.[10] Indeed, we have not seen the same kinds of changes regarding the stigmatization of self-injury that we have for many other mental health difficulties. There are many reasons for this. For instance, by its very nature, self-injury is a deliberate behavior in which one injures themselves and which can result in visible marks in the form of injuries and potential scarring. Far too many people in society therefore have difficulty comprehending *why* a person would intentionally injure themselves, which can provoke negative and otherwise unhelpful attitudes, reactions, assumptions, and stereotypes.[10]

As discussed earlier in this book, stigma in the context of self-injury is widespread, with innumerable accounts of stigma in lay, educational, and healthcare settings.[11-16] Cognizant of this stigma, people with lived experience of self-injury are understandably reluctant—and often very much unwilling—to share their experiences or seek needed support and care.[16,17] Furthermore, there is reason to believe that stigma may also apply to the research context, as people with lived experience of self-injury are seldom involved in the research beyond the role of participant.[1]

Another barrier to greater inclusion of lived experience voices may stem from people's views of individuals who self-injure. Indeed, individuals who self-injure may be deemed vulnerable; as such, their involvement in research or other enterprises may be seen as risky.[18] For instance, a study may ask participants to engage in tasks that induce stress (or other difficult emotional states) or involve exposure to material that might be upsetting or triggering (e.g., viewing images related to self-injury). Adding to this are long-standing views that by taking part in research on self-injury, individuals may be more apt to self-injure.[1,18] Collectively, these concerns may make researchers (and others) cautious about involving individuals who self-injure beyond the conventional position of research participant. Although research can indeed carry some level of risk, concerns about research participation provoking self-injury (also referred to as iatrogenic risk) has been subject to investigation, with findings indicating that people do *not* report greater self-injury engagement immediately—or even days—after taking part in self-injury research.[19]

In sum, the formal inclusion of people with lived experience in research and other activities (e.g., service delivery) are comparably lagging versus other areas (e.g., depression, eating disorders). We argue that this lack of representation is not only a missed opportunity but also a hindrance to advancing the field.[1] By working toward greater inclusion of people with lived experience, the field of self-injury would ostensibly be better positioned to: (a) enhance the development, conducting, and dissemination of research; (b) tailor research to meet people's needs; (c) increase self-injury awareness and address its stigmatization; and (d) inspire hope, facilitate support seeking, and improve service delivery. Formal inclusion of lived experience voices must therefore be prioritized given its promise to effect meaningful, needed, and lasting change.[1]

WHY LIVED EXPERIENCE VOICES ARE NEEDED

At a basic level, people with lived experience of self-injury are often quite willing to take on a multitude of roles in the field. For instance, researchers have demonstrated that many individuals who self-injure take part in research for altruistic and self-motivated reasons, including to advance knowledge and help others.[1,20] Likewise, people often use social media and other online platforms (e.g., The Mighty, podcasts) to discuss shared concerns, bring people together, offer support, and to increase awareness of self-injury.[1,21-23]

More intentional involvement of people with lived experience in the process of research can help allow for *true* priority-driven research—that is, research which ensures people's primary concerns are addressed. This does not mean, of course, that the research produced to date has not significantly advanced what we know about self-injury or that similar kinds of research should be ceased moving forward. Rather, we contend that by bringing people with lived experience into *all* stages of the process of research, we can bolster how we understand and address self-injury. In other words, people's formal inclusion in research represents a vital means of *maximizing* the nature and impact of research conducted. For example, consideration of lived experience views can help address many outstanding issues in our field. This includes (but is no way confined to): understanding what thwarts and leads to support-seeking, how to best serve and support people when they engage with mental health services, how to work toward greater inclusion and representation of diverse experience, how to optimize training for service deliverers, how to maximize antistigma efforts, and how to foster resilience and recovery.

To meet these and other research aims, the person-centered approach woven throughout this book is essential. As mentioned in Chapter 5, how we talk about self-injury and refer to people with lived experience matters. Thus, avoidance of words and framings that label a person (e.g., "self-injurer") or that are value laden (e.g., referring to self-injury as "maladaptive") are pejorative and can be quite hurtful for people on the receiving end.[1,24–27] Hence, their (often inadvertent) presence in research settings may thwart the very purpose driving the research. Being mindful of the impact of language from the outset helps to avoid such occurrences (e.g., during recruitment, when interacting with a participant). This has the benefit of people being more likely to have a positive experience when taking part in research, perhaps incentivizing them to take part in future studies or perhaps take on their own advocacy-like roles.

Although concerns about involvement in self-injury research (e.g., iatrogenic effects) may have historically impeded the formal inclusion of people with lived experience in the research process, evidence points to several benefits for people who have self-injured when taking part in research.[1] For example, many people report that their research participation permits reflection and, in turn, more understanding about their own experience with self-injury.[28] Additionally, taking part in research may provide a platform on which to share (at least part of) one's story.[1] In our own work, we have heard from innumerable people that being able to share parts of their experience in a research context (e.g., in an interview) can be validating, cathartic, and ultimately quite helpful. This is in line with a vast literature on mental illness suggesting that sharing one's experience with another can help to decrease self-stigma, enhance interpersonal relationships, and spur professional help-seeking.[29] Along these lines, participating in self-injury research can also be empowering and have positive effects on self-esteem, self-confidence, and a person's sense of meaning.[20] For individuals who elect to pursue leadership roles in self-injury research, this may be especially relevant and motivating.[1]

In the context of service provision and associated clinical work (e.g., assessment), drawing on lived experience perspectives can help ensure that people's needs are fully met by appropriately tailoring the nature of the services offered.[1,30] As discussed in Chapter 11 on recovery, no two people's experiences with self-injury are identical.[2] Thus, while it is likely that specific approaches (e.g., dialectical behavior therapy to enhance distress tolerance) are bound to be helpful for large numbers of individuals, avoiding generalizations about the utility of any one approach for *all* people is important. A person-centered approach takes into account individual differences and is therefore well-suited to meeting people's diverse needs.[30] This is also in keeping with calls from the field[1,30] and content from our prior chapters.

Attending to lived experience perspectives also represents a key component of effective outreach and advocacy.[1] One part of this is tackling stigma. Congruent with efforts to combat stigma associated with broader mental health difficulties,[7-9] lived experience voices are vital to meeting these critical aims in the context of self-injury.[4] In particular, "contact-based" efforts in which people with lived experience are directly involved in the changing of public attitudes of, and discourses about, self-injury are likely to be fruitful as they have the twofold benefit of addressing stigma while concurrently empowering people with lived experience.[4,7-9,31,32] Although calls have been made for participatory approaches to tackle the stigmatization of self-injury[1,4] they have not yet translated to action.

As strides are made in the field to include more lived experience voices, it will be important to adopt a forward-thinking approach to these initiatives. Notably, opportunities need to be explicitly made available for people with lived experience to undertake a range of advocacy roles. This should include and not be limited to research positions, service and related decision-making roles, antistigma work, and leadership positions. In doing so, lived experience perspectives can be sustainably incorporated throughout the field, which can work to inspire future generations to seek these roles.[1,3]

Finally, in any work involving lived experience considerations, we encourage readers to employ a wide lens when thinking about what lived experience means. Certainly, much of the discussion so far emphasizes the inclusion of people who, themselves, have self-injured. As discussed in previous chapters, however, support people can also play key roles in the context of understanding and addressing self-injury. This includes school professionals, mental health professionals, families— anyone who knows someone or who has worked with someone who has lived experience of self-injury. By adopting a multifaceted view of lived experience, we will be much better equipped to meet the critical aims noted in this chapter.

LIVED EXPERIENCE RESEARCH: CURRENT STATE OF THE FIELD

A scan of the extant literature indicates that researchers have largely sought to identify factors that associate with the onset of self-injury, those linked with its repetition, and differences between people who do and do not self-injure. In other words, much of the published research has focused on ascertaining self-injury correlates and risk factors. Ultimately, these efforts have provided insight into why people engage in self-injury, therefore establishing a much-needed knowledge base in the field. Missing from this, however, is a deeper appreciation and comprehension of what it means to self-injure—notably, from the vantage point of people with lived experience.

Fostering a deeper understanding of the experience of self-injury goes beyond (but may still at times include) identification of specific risk or maintaining factors. For instance, this could involve more qualitative, bottom-up approaches. On the next few pages, we therefore summarize recent efforts in this burgeoning line of work that focused on understanding: how self-injury is conceptualized and the extent to which it ought to be considered in the diagnostic nomenclature; understanding self-injury recovery; how disclosures are navigated; and how stigma is experienced. Collectively, and in line with the main tenet of this book, these efforts have underscored the centrality of a person-centered approach to understanding self-injury.

Self-Injury as a Mental Disorder

As mentioned in Chapter 1, self-injury was included in the fifth iteration of the *Diagnostic and Statistical Manual for Mental Disorders* (DSM).[33] Preceding this was significant debate across several disciplines about whether self-injury should be considered as a mental disorder.[34,35] A fundamental part of this polemic has been at what point one's self-injury engagement should be rendered "pathological." To address this, researchers have recently examined how clinicians and researchers in the field conceptualize self-injury.[36] Interestingly, but perhaps not surprisingly, findings from this study highlighted much disagreement about what constituted self-injury. Of note was the frequency criterion used in the proposed criteria for Non-Suicidal Self-Injury Disorder, which stipulates that a person would need to self-injure on 5 or more days in the past 12 months for the criterion to be met.[35] Many viewed this as too low a threshold both in terms of the number of times one self-injures and the period over which it occurs. This is consistent with several papers,[37–40] including a recent study in which it was suggested that focusing on the last month (versus year) may be a more clinically meaningful timeframe to consider.[40]

While it is certainly important to ask researchers and clinicians about the prospect of self-injury as a standalone diagnosis, ascertaining the views of people with lived experience is also needed. To this end, our team conducted a study a few years ago in which we asked people with lived experience what they thought about the possibility of self-injury being a formal mental disorder.[41] Interestingly, participants indicated mixed views. On the one hand, some people discussed potential benefits of this prospect; for example, they shared that including self-injury as a diagnostic category would validate their experience, enhance research in the field, and improve self-injury intervention. On the other hand, participants also expressed trepidation that the inclusion of self-injury in the diagnostic nomenclature could worsen stigma and that too much focus on self-injury itself would dismiss concerns underlying and associated with their self-injury engagement (e.g., underlying adversities). As such, should self-injury eventually be incorporated in the DSM, clinicians must endeavor to understand the views and concerns of clients who may receive such a diagnosis. Doing so is key to ensuring effective and collaborative engagement in the therapeutic process.

Understanding Recovery

In many ways, the very foundation of the person-centered model of recovery presented in Chapter 11 comes from lived experience views—this includes research we have conducted as well as that from others in the field. For example, in one of our studies, we asked people about their views on what recovery means to them and what it involves.[42] When reading what people shared, it became abundantly clear that individuals hold diverse and nuanced views about what constitutes recovery. Notably, they highlighted that recovery is a complex and nonlinear process that varies across individuals. They also shared that recovery may mean that urges to self-injure do not fully dissipate (but may lessen in intensity) and that through one's recovery journey, resilience and strength can be cultivated. In another one of our studies involving adolescents, participants discussed how recovery meant an absence of urges to self-injure.[43] They also discussed having much ambivalence about engaging in self-injury, citing continued thoughts about self-injury as well as urges to hurt themselves, while also expressing that they had stopped self-injury, or liked to think they had stopped. While a fulsome presentation of these and other studies is incorporated in our recovery model (Chapter 11), these collective insights are illustrative of the value and resultant contributions of intentionally working to understand people's lived experience views.

Looking ahead, we believe that the more we draw on people's lived experience of recovery, the better positioned the field will be to help individuals work toward recovery in a way that works for them; in turn, this can result in more positive treatment experiences and outcomes. Supporting this view are the countless positive anecdotes we have heard when presenting our framework to both people who have lived experience and clinicians who work with them. Indeed, people have reported feeling validated and hopeful with the formal acknowledgment that recovery comprises far more than just stopping self-injury. Of course, a next step in this area will be to apply the model more formally and examine its overall utility.

Navigating Disclosures

The salience of disclosure for many individuals with lived experience of self-injury cannot be overstated. Indeed, the choice to share one's self-injury experience with another person can be quite difficult. For reasons that include but go beyond stigma, far too many individuals who have self-injured opt to hide their behavior from others; in many cases, people feel as though they have no choice but to hide self-injury. If self-injury is disclosed, people typically turn to close others such as friends or family rather than discussing their experience with a health or mental health professional.[44]

Researchers have found that sharing one's self-injury experience in informal contexts, such as with family, may represent a steppingstone in the process of accessing professional support.[20] Nonetheless, people with lived experience cite shame, self- and anticipated stigma, and worry about burdening others as major impediments to disclosure.[17,44,45] These concerns are understandable. They are also grounded in data. Indeed, a review of the literature concerning disclosure indicated that people frequently experience negative and otherwise unhelpful reactions from others in disclosure contexts.[44] Further, there is a greater likelihood of people disclosing self-injury when their injuries warrant medical attention or when they experience suicidal thinking.[46] Given these contextual considerations, these disclosures may not necessarily signal a deliberate decision to share one's experience; rather, these disclosures may stem from a particular need (e.g., medical care for injuries, to navigate a crisis) versus a choice to share one's experience.

When thinking about self-injury disclosures, it is important to account for the many ways they can manifest. Indeed, while much of the discussion thus far involves—at least to some degree—voluntary disclosure, not all disclosures occur in this way. In some cases, individuals may experience involuntary, or even forced disclosure. For instance, people who have visible scarring from self-injury may be asked about their scars, which can result in an unexpected, and perhaps unwanted, disclosure. As another example, a person's self-injury may be shared with a third party (e.g., a concerned friend may confide to someone if they are worried about their friend's self-injury). These kinds of involuntary disclosures (or discoveries) are ostensibly more difficult for individuals with lived experience due to a lack of readiness and control over the nature of the disclosure, including to whom one's experience is "disclosed."

It would then follow that disclosure and its many permutations warrant greater research consideration, including within but not exclusive to a recovery context. This line of work must therefore draw on people's lived experience, with recognition that this is broadly defined. In this way, such work should involve people who self-injure along with the other individuals involved in disclosure contexts. This kind of work will help elucidate how people navigate disclosures, how all people involved are impacted, and, critically, how we can best support individuals with lived experience in these contexts.

Stigma

At this point of the book, it should be clear that self-injury stigma is significant and sweeping in impact.[11] Research involving lived experience views has thus been helpful in beginning to inform how we understand such stigma. For example, it has been shown that self-inflicted injuries bring about greater stigma than injuries that are unintentional.[47] Other research has indicated that people may be more dismissive of individuals when they disclose their self-injury due to endorsement of particular stereotypes (e.g., seeing self-injury as attention seeking).[48] Consistent with this, people have told us that shame represents a major hurdle to reaching out to others as they are concerned about how people will react.[17]

In thinking about the roles that people can play in the field, stigma may emerge as especially relevant when people with lived experience are themselves researchers and/or clinicians. For researchers, conducting self-relevant research (often dismissively referred to as "me-search") is often viewed negatively; this includes views that this kind of research ought to be avoided, that it is somehow selfish (e.g., it primarily concerns one's own experience), that it lacks rigor and credibility, and that it is inherently biased.[49-51] Despite the pervasiveness of these attitudes, we note there are notable benefits associated with people who have lived experience leading research on topics of self-relevance. For example, this may permit topics that may otherwise go overlooked to gain needed research attention. This kind of research can also translate to priority-driven efforts that meet the needs of people who have lived experience. Outside of this, having people with lived experience in established research positions can inspire other individuals to pursue similar roles, including key mentorship roles (e.g., in graduate programs).[1,3,51]

For clinicians with lived experience (including trainees), there may be worry that any form of disclosure may thwart their career trajectory, perhaps by disqualifying them from admission to professional programs, or resulting in perceptions that they are incompetent or insufficiently divorced from their own experience to be an effective clinician.[51] These examples of manifested stigma may deter otherwise excellent clinicians from seeking positions in which they could provide meaningful support to others. As such, it will be important to engage in efforts to ensure that up-and-coming clinicians are not thwarted in their pursuit of their career ambitions. Growing efforts in this area that work to challenge unhelpful views that impede people from seeking these roles are bound to be useful moving forward.[49-51]

Finally, lived experience insights have been instrumental in helping to understand how language may be a source of stigma (see Chapter 5 for more details). For example, we recently published a study in which we sought to elicit what kinds of words and phrasings people in the field of self-injury used and what they saw as appropriate when referring to self-injury and people with lived experience.[27] Results indicated that people with lived experience, in contrast to individuals who primarily identify as researchers and clinicians, differed in a few ways with respect to the appropriateness of certain terms. At the same time, we also found some common ground with respect to language use. For instance, researchers and clinicians were less likely to use terms that referenced individuals with lived experience (e.g., people with a history of self-injury) but tended to concur that terms like "manipulative" should not be used. Informed by these results, we called on researchers and clinicians to reflect on and consider the nature of language they use given the potential impact it may have on people with lived experience.

ADOPTING A PERSON-CENTERED APPROACH

Bringing all these considerations together, we argue for a person-centered approach to understand an individual's experience of self-injury—one that explicitly acknowledges that each person is an expert in their *own* story, and people's stories will be different. Making assumptions about why someone self-injures, and what their experience is like, only mutes their story, minimizes the potential for rapport, and risks invalidating that experience. For individuals who already feel misunderstood and isolated, this only exacerbates these feelings, and further silences them. In moving our understanding of self-injury forward, it is imperative to continue *actively* listening to individuals with lived experience of self-injury and make concerted efforts to involve them in all phases of research, practice, and outreach.[1] We therefore draw readers' attention to the next section, which offers practical strategies in this regard.

PRACTICAL APPLICATIONS

When incorporating a person-centered approach that emphasizes lived experience views in research, clinical work, and outreach, several ethical challenges may emerge. Thus, in what follows we highlight what these are and offer solutions to address them. Although we have partitioned the remainder of the chapter along the domains of research, clinical work, and outreach, we recognize that people frequently have simultaneous roles in more than one (or even all) of these spaces.

Research

Individuals with lived experience possess expertise in the experience of self-injury and can provide insights conducive to advancing our collective understanding of self-injury.[1] As described earlier, much of the work in this area to date has mostly relied on asking people who have self-injured about their lived experience but in their role as research participants. Beyond the utility this approach affords (e.g., offering novel perspectives on self-injury recovery), these lines of inquiry could be enriched by not only eliciting lived experience views in later stages of research (i.e., data collection) but also in earlier research stages.

For example, during the initial phases of research, individuals with lived experience can offer helpful views on the focus of research by helping to inform and shape research agendas and questions. One particular kind of research that has relevance in this regard is participatory action research.[52] In general, participatory action research draws on an array of methodologies that directly involve people with lived experience at *all* research stages; hence, individuals take part in the planning, implementation, and dissemination of research.[53-59] Of course, when carrying out this kind of work, several ethical considerations will need to be made. For instance, given the level of people's involvement, it would be important that any such undertaking involve appropriate compensation for people's time and expertise (especially if they are asked to devote time that takes away from employment or their families). Furthermore, it would be important to ensure that participants are provided with resources. These could be used should any aspect of their involvement provoke emotional upset, such as when very difficult topics (e.g., experiencing a stigmatizing or hurtful reaction during a disclosure) are addressed. In this way, drawing on some of the established recommendations for ethically conducting research on self-injury may be warranted.[18]

Participatory-based research often focuses on concerns that are underrepresented, stigmatized, or misunderstood, thereby frequently involving people who are marginalized in society.[53-59] In this way, it may have relevance to self-injury (e.g., tackling stigma).[4] Moreover, when implemented and having people take part in all phases of research, evidence shows that participatory-based research has several benefits for people involved. For example, there are reports that involvement in participatory action research can be empowering and help individuals to reclaim voice when they previously felt silenced.[55,56,58,59] Given this, researchers have called for the use of these methodologies in self-injury research.[4] To date, however, such efforts are scant. Indeed, when reviewing the literature, we identified less than a handful of participatory action research studies.[60-61]

There are likely many reasons to explain the paucity of participatory action research studies in the self-injury field, including the barriers outlined earlier (e.g., stigma, concern about iatrogenic effects). At a broader level, however, is psychology's historical reliance on dominant positivist paradigms.[62] These paradigms comprise the view that knowledge about a phenomenon can only be ascertained if it can be reduced to, and thus measured as, an observable experience; it also involves the notion that researchers must remain objective and thus separate from their research.[63] Hence, certain kinds of research (e.g., experimental methods) have been preferred over qualitative approaches to research, which would include participatory action research and related methods situating lived experience at the forefront.

Building on this, and likely contributing to hesitancy (and perhaps resistance) for the inclusion of people with lived experience in the process of research are concerns about a lack of objectivity that may be seen as missing from research conducted by individuals with lived experience, including self-relevant research described earlier. Through this lens, subjectivity would be viewed as a major drawback to rigorous, high-quality study as "good" research must be (or at least strive to be) fully objective. We counter this perspective by suggesting that no research can be truly, and completely, objective. We contend that people's past experiences, including their theoretical and epistemological orientations, are inevitably tied to their approach to research—whether it be qualitative or quantitative, based on personal experience or not. To this end, one cannot fully divorce subjectivity from their approach to research and thus their pursuit of knowledge.

There is arguably much to be learned from a more lived-experience approach to research. Harkening back to participatory action research, a major reason these methods are beneficial is the *process* of research itself. In many qualitative research approaches and the philosophies that underpin them, a main focus is on the process of the research.[64] The same goes for participatory action research and the impact of engagement in the research process.[52–59] Beyond the process of research, however, is also the knowledge gleaned through research that centers people's experiences. In line with sentiments from others[65] there is therefore value in moving beyond more traditional and historically dominant paradigms and implementing others.[66]

Although there are barriers to undertaking lived experience research, we are seeing a shift in recent years of more and more researchers seeking to understand how people navigate their self-injury experience. And while these efforts are important, many of the studies to date are narrow in terms of which stories are represented. Much like a significant portion of quantitative work, much of work examining lived experience of self-injury involves white, cis-gendered women from university settings. Accordingly, the extent to which findings from these studies apply to more diverse groups is limited. It is therefore incumbent on researchers to work toward greater inclusion and diversity in the voices elevated through research.

In an effort to work toward more inclusion and greater representation in the stories shared through research, however, unique ethical considerations may again surface. For instance, ensuring participants have safe, trauma-informed spaces to share their stories would be critical; appropriate reimbursement would also be important. As needed, learning from relevant literatures, seeking resources, and, as appropriate, consulting with individuals from diverse backgrounds to ensure that questions are being asked in a sensitive manner can work to mitigate against the potential for aspects of the project to move forward in ways that are inappropriate or insensitive to people's backgrounds.

Clinical Work and Applications

As mentioned earlier in the book, a person-centered approach has relevance in clinical contexts and in fostering recovery. Central to this is the principle that no two individuals are identical when it comes to their experience of self-injury.[2,30] Therefore, a collaborative, bottom-up, and flexible clinical approach that endeavors to elicit and understand a person's story and experience with self-injury is recommended. This allows clinicians to better develop a formulation that understands an individual's unique challenges *and* strengths instead of relying on a single framework (e.g., emotion regulation) or intervention (e.g., cognitive behavior therapy). Adopting such a holistic approach also has the benefit of not spending too much focus on self-injury, which is a concern some individuals have.[30,41] Collectively, attention to these considerations in the context of clinical work can help increase the likelihood that someone will be engaged and motivated throughout the therapeutic process.

Consistent with this is checking in with the individual at different time points to elicit their views, goals, and concerns. This is especially important as these factors may very well change over the course of recovery. Deferring to these person-centered considerations also avoids inadvertently pushing a particular conception of what recovery should look like. Of course, this does not mean that a clinician takes a backseat to the point they are not engaged; we are also not implying that clinicians refrain from offering clinically relevant observations or views (e.g., if a client's self-injury is increasing in severity, this should still be discussed). Rather, a person-centered approach means finding a balance that allows space for the above considerations while also communicating clinically germane views and concerns in a compassionate manner. This is done while remaining situated within the context of a client's broader experience.

Finally, it is important to bear in mind that individuals may hold differing views on traditional clinical approaches. In some instances, there may be structural or systemic considerations that make it harder for some groups to even access treatment (e.g., among Black, Indigenous, and People of Color, as well as LGBTQ+ individuals, among whom rates of NSSI are elevated). More research is thus needed to shed light on issues of accessibility and appropriateness of different treatment modalities for people from diverse and marginalized backgrounds (including the intersection of several identities). Nevertheless, building awareness about racial trauma and oppression and the impact this has on people is important. Hence, clinicians are encouraged to seek consultation, knowledge, and training to ensure a trauma-informed and culturally humble and competent approach when working with diverse clients. Trauma-informed and culturally aware providers are essential to providing support to individuals with marginalized identities. As we look to progress the broader clinical field, working to ensure equal opportunity and training to individuals from marginalized backgrounds should also be prioritized.

Outreach Applications

In the last part of this chapter, we address how lived experience views are pivotal to successful outreach initiatives. Akin to what was described earlier for effective antistigma efforts (also see Chapter 4), outreach and advocacy initiatives should similarly position lived experience stories as a potent vehicle not only to combat stigma but also to increase awareness and understanding.[4] Beyond sharing of people's experiences, it would be important to ensure these individuals help to inform and plan these initiatives, especially if their story is to be used in some capacity. Further, and like ethically conducted research, appropriate compensation would again be an essential consideration.

When embarking on outreach projects, several potential concerns merit discussion. Often, campaigns and other events tend to draw on experiences in which people share their story of recovery. No doubt such stories are important and much needed. They can inspire hope and validate other individuals' experiences. At the same time, it would be important that shared stories do not dismiss or overlook the difficulties that many people will encounter. For example, the process of recovery is nonlinear, and setbacks or difficulties are more the norm than exception within one's recovery journey;[2] thus sole focus on recovery "outcomes" that gloss over some of these common experiences may not fully resonate with many people and may give a false impression of what recovery ought to look like.

When researchers and clinicians are invited to speak at events, it is not uncommon for them to be financially compensated. Yet, this may not be typical practice when individuals with lived experience are invited, unless they are also a researcher and/or clinician. Ensuring that *all* speakers are appropriately compensated is therefore important from an ethical standpoint. It ensures that advocates—in particular, if they do not occupy a higher status role in the field—are not taken for granted or assumed to be willing to take part in events at no cost. Ensuring individuals are compensated also works to increase the diversity of perspectives offered in public outreach. Diversifying the nature of stories heard in outreach initiatives, including those that have been more historically marginalized, reduces the chances that a small number of experiences will overshadow others (e.g., only seeking a specific narrative or self-injury experience, only inviting presenters from specific demographic backgrounds). In line with a person-centered approach, advocacy efforts must strive to incorporate stories that are not part of the mainstream. To accomplish this, it will be important to engage in efforts to reach out to all segments of society and to be willing to confront and engage in dialogue about topics that may be challenging in the process (e.g., systemic racism, colonization, oppression).

Much as with research, there are bound to be concerns about the impact of outreach work amongst advocates (e.g., concern about a speaker feeling vulnerable or that their participation will provoke upset). In some cases, it might be helpful to offer people a safe space to enhance their comfort when sharing parts of their experience (e.g., eliciting and respecting their concerns or wishes about a particular event). In concert with this is ensuring appropriate and relevant resources and support are available for individual advocates as well as members of the audience (who may also be impacted in outreach events). Putting these safeguards in place can limit the potential impact of any content or knowledge shared (e.g., a distressing part of one's story). Finally, when working with individuals in the context of advocacy and outreach, ensuring that individuals are not tokenized is imperative. Hence, true person-centered approaches would work to ensure that all advocates are viewed holistically—as unique individuals with full lives, experiences, and emotions.

SUMMARY

Across various disciplines, there have been calls and initiatives to formally involve people with lived experience of mental health difficulties. Although similar efforts have emerged to some degree for self-injury, we believe much more can and must be done to propel research, clinical, and outreach work. Evidence for the utility of such work can be seen through the content woven throughout this book.

Therefore, by reflecting on the content of this chapter, and embracing a person-centered approach, it is our hope that readers will be better equipped to take on advocacy roles and pursue work in any or all the areas addressed here. Indeed, the only question remaining when adopting a person-centered approach to advance self-injury research, clinical practice, and outreach is: *how can we not?*

Through our collective experience working with countless individuals with lived experience in research, clinical, and outreach capacities, it became increasingly and abundantly clear that notwithstanding tremendous advances in our understanding of self-injury over the years, a *true* person-centered approach was conspicuously absent. Indeed, the bulk of the literature has been dominated by deficit-based approaches that emphasize what individuals with lived experience do not have or should obtain. Along these lines, and although largely inadvertent, there are innumerable examples of unhelpful language that may reduce individuals to a behavior (e.g., self-injurers) or place value on how they are functioning (e.g., morbid form of self-help or a maladaptive coping). Furthermore, due to the favorability of certain ways of conducting research and advancing knowledge, much of what has been written may unintentionally lead to assumptions about homogeneity among groups of individuals with lived experience. For people with lived experience, this can lead to a perception of exclusion and a sense of not feeling understood.

There is no doubt that our understanding of self-injury would not be where it is today without the significant strides made over the past 20 or so years. Likewise, without this work, we would not have been able to have written his book. Nevertheless, through our own experience, and following many discussions with people who have self-injured, it became evident that greater attention to people's lived experience was needed. Central to this was the need for explicit recognition that every individual's experience of self-injury is unique. This is not to say there are not similarities across people's experiences. There are. Yet, we maintain that to fully and authentically appreciate a person's experience of self-injury, a paradigm shift is needed—one that centers a person's distinct set of experiences and does so devoid of judgment and preconception. Accordingly, the person-centered approach threaded throughout this book challenges the canonical deficit-based models of self-injury and ways of approaching the field. In doing so, we intentionally and explicitly recognize the inner fortitude, perseverance, and resilience that all people with lived experience possess.

We believe readers will not only have a foundational understanding of self-injury but ultimately a deeper and more compassionate appreciation of people's experience of self-injury upon reading this book. Hence, by drawing on the person-centered framework woven throughout the book, readers will be poised to adopt this approach when embarking on their own work in the field—irrespecitve of which role (or roles) this entails. To this end, a key first step is understanding the complexities and impact of the stigmatization of self-injury is critical. In a similar manner, cognizance of the language one uses—and that is used by others—is vital for everyone when writing or talking about self-injury. This is especially important when talking with (and not to) people with lived experience.

For school professionals, a person-centered approach can work to inform and enhance how students who self-injure are approached, heard, and supported. In a similar vein, we hope that parents and caregivers of youth who self-injure will feel more equipped and confident in their understanding of their child's self-injury and thus be better able to offer support. Indeed, for all individuals who play key support roles, the content articulated in the book, including how to navigate discussions about self-injury, is conducive to facilitating a deeper and more compassionate understanding of a person's experience with self-injury. Building on this, for clinicians and trainees, we hope that our person-centered model of recovery allows for an even more comprehensive understanding of their clients' experiences and that by drawing on this, they will be able to incorporate person-centered considerations that harness and promote people's strengths and underlying resilience. Finally, for researchers, it is our intent that the content presented throughout this book ignites new lines of inquiry, dialogue about conducting research, and inclusion of people with lived experience throughout the process of research.

The time has come to challenge the status quo. To advance our field—in research, clinical, and outreach capacities—we need to not just adopt but also advocate for a person-centered approach. It is incumbent on us all to do this. Certainly, there may be obstacles along the way. However, we contend that the costs of not doing so far outweighs the work needed to overcome these challenges. We therefore hope, that upon reading our book, readers will be more inspired and hopeful in their work supporting individuals who engage in self-injury. Embracing a person-centered approach allows for all of us to become advocates for individuals with lived experience. It is our hope that readers will be emboldened in this regard. By using a person-centered approach, we will be ideally positioned to propel the field in the domains of research, clinical work, and outreach. Ultimately, this can work to cultivate and sustain meaningful and lasting change in the lives of people with lived experience of self-injury.

Chapter 1

1. International Society for the Study of Self-Injury. (2018). *About self injury*. Retrieved July 25, 2021, from https://itriples. org/category/about-self-injury/

2. Swannell, S. V., Martin, G. E., Page, A., Hasking, P., & St John, N. J. (2014). Prevalence of nonsuicidal self-injury in nonclinical samples: Systematic review, meta-analysis and meta-regression. *Suicide and Life-Threatening Behavior, 44*(3), 273–303.

3. Klonsky, E. D., & Muehlenkamp, J. J. (2007). Self-injury: A research review for the practitioner. *Journal of Clinical Psychology, 63*(11), 1045–1056.

4. Web of Science. (2021). www.webofknowledge.com (accessed August 14, 2021).

5. Lewis, S. P., & Heath, N. L. (2015). Nonsuicidal self-injury among youth. *Journal of Pediatrics, 166*(3), 526–530.

6. Glenn, C. R., & Klonsky, E. D. (2013). Nonsuicidal self-injury disorder: An empirical investigation in adolescent psychiatric patients. *Journal of Clinical Child and Adolescent Psychology, 42*(4), 496–507.

7. Muehlenkamp, J. J., Ertelt, T. W., Miller, A. L., & Claes, L. (2011). Borderline personality symptoms differentiate non-suicidal and suicidal self-injury in ethnically diverse adolescent outpatients. *Journal of Child Psychology and Psychiatry, 52*(2), 148–155.

8. Gandhi, A., Luyckx, K., Baetens, I., Kiekens, G., Sleuwaegen, E., Berens, A., . . . Claes, L. (2018). Age of onset of non-suicidal self-injury in Dutch-speaking adolescents and emerging adults: An event history analysis of pooled data. *Comprehensive Psychiatry, 80*, 170–178.

9. Martin, G., Swannell, S. V., Hazell, P. L., Harrison, J. E., & Taylor, A. W. (2010). Self-injury in Australia: A community survey. *Medical Journal of Australia, 193*(9), 506–510.

10. Muehlenkamp, J. J., Claes, L., Havertape, L., & Plener, P. L. (2012). International prevalence of adolescent non-suicidal self-injury and deliberate self-harm. *Child and Adolescent Psychiatry and Mental Health, 6*(1), 1–9.

11. Wester, K., Trepal, H., & King, K. (2018). Nonsuicidal self-injury: Increased prevalence in engagement. *Suicide and Life-Threatening Behavior, 48*(6), 690–698.

12. Lewis, S. P., Heath, N. L., Hasking, P. A., Whitlock, J. L., Wilson, M. S., & Plener, P. L. (2019). Addressing self-injury on college campuses: Institutional recommendations. *Journal of College Counseling, 22*(1), 70–82.

13. Klonsky, E. D. (2011). Non-suicidal self-injury in United States adults: Prevalence, sociodemographics, topography and functions. *Psychological Medicine, 41*(9), 1981–1986.

14. Liu, R. T. (2021). The epidemiology of non-suicidal self-injury: Lifetime prevalence, sociodemographic and clinical correlates, and treatment use in a nationally representative sample of adults in England. *Psychological Medicine,* 1–9. https://doi.org/10.1017/S003329172100146X

15. Barrocas, A. L., Hankin, B. L., Young, J. F., & Abela, J. R. (2012). Rates of nonsuicidal self-injury in youth: Age, sex, and behavioral methods in a community sample. *Pediatrics, 130*(1), 39–45.

16. Darche, M. A. (1990). Psychological factors differentiating self-mutilating and non-self-mutilating adolescent inpatient females. *The Psychiatric Hospital, 21,* 31–35.

17. DiClemente, R. J., Ponton, L. E., & Hartley, D. (1991). Prevalence and correlates of cutting behavior: Risk for HIV transmission. *Journal of the American Academy of Child and Adolescent Psychiatry, 30,* 735–739.

18. Pérez, S., Marco, J. H., & Cañabate, M. (2018). Non-suicidal self-injury in patients with eating disorders: Prevalence, forms, functions, and body image correlates. *Comprehensive Psychiatry, 84,* 32–38.

19. Cucchi, A., Ryan, D., Konstantakopoulos, G., Stroumpa, S., Kaçar, A. Ş., Renshaw, S., . . . Kravariti, E. (2016). Lifetime prevalence of non-suicidal self-injury in patients with eating disorders: A systematic review and meta-analysis. *Psychological Medicine, 46*(7), 1345–1358.

20. Hauber, K., Boon, A., & Vermeiren, R. (2019). Non-suicidal self-injury in clinical practice. *Frontiers in Psychology, 10,* 502.

21. Gholamrezaei, M., De Stefano, J., & Heath, N. L. (2017). Nonsuicidal self-injury across cultures and ethnic and racial minorities: A review. *International Journal of Psychology, 52*(4), 316–326.

22. Rojas-Velasquez, D. A., Pluhar, E. I., Burns, P. A., & Burton, E. T. (2021). Nonsuicidal self-injury among African American and Hispanic adolescents and young adults: A systematic review. *Prevention Science, 22*(3), 367–377.

23. Victor, S. E., Muehlenkamp, J. J., Hayes, N. A., Lengel, G. J., Styer, D. M., & Washburn, J. J. (2018). Characterizing gender differences in nonsuicidal self-injury: Evidence from a large clinical sample of adolescents and adults. *Comprehensive Psychiatry, 82,* 53–60.

24. Whitlock, J., Muehlenkamp, J., Purington, A., Eckenrode, J., Barreira, P., Baral Abrams, G., . . . Knox, K. (2011). Nonsuicidal self-injury in a college population: General trends and sex differences. *Journal of American College Health, 59*(8), 691–698.

25. Whitlock, J., Eckenrode, J., & Silverman, D. (2006). Self-injurious behaviors in a college population. *Pediatrics, 117*(6), 1939–1948.

26. Dolan, I. J., Strauss, P., Winter, S., & Lin, A. (2020). Misgendering and experiences of stigma in health care settings for transgender people. *Medical Journal of Australia, 212*(4), 150–151.

27. Batejan, K. L., Jarvi, S. M., & Swenson, L. P. (2015). Sexual orientation and non-suicidal self-injury: A meta-analytic review. *Archives of Suicide Research, 19*(2), 131–150.

28. Jackman, K. B., Dolezal, C., Levin, B., Honig, J. C., & Bockting, W. O. (2018). Stigma, gender dysphoria, and nonsuicidal self-injury in a community sample of transgender individuals. *Psychiatry Research, 269,* 602–609.

29. Liu, R. T., Sheehan, A. E., Walsh, R. F., Sanzari, C. M., Cheek, S. M., & Hernandez, E. M. (2019). Prevalence and correlates of non-suicidal self-injury among lesbian, gay, bisexual, and transgender individuals: A systematic review and meta-analysis. *Clinical Psychology Review, 74,* 101783.

30. Marshall, E., Claes, L., Bouman, W. P., Witcomb, G. L., & Arcelus, J. (2016). Non-suicidal self-injury and suicidality in trans people: A systematic review of the literature. *International Review of Psychiatry, 28*(1), 58–69.

31. Strauss, P., Cook, A., Winter, S., Watson, V., Toussaint, D. W., & Lin, A. (2020). Associations between negative life experiences and the mental health of trans and gender diverse young people in Australia: Findings from trans pathways. *Psychological Medicine, 50*(5), 808–817.

32. Nock, M. K. (2010). Self-injury. *Annual Review of Clinical Psychology, 6,* 339–363.

33. Nock, M. K. (Ed.). (2014). *The Oxford handbook of suicide and self-injury.* Oxford University Press.

34. Klonsky, E. D., Muehlenkamp, J., Lewis, S. P., & Walsh, B. (2011). *Nonsuicidal self-injury* (Vol. 22). Hogrefe Publishing.

35. Washburn, J. J. (Ed.). (2019). *Nonsuicidal self-injury: Advances in research and practice.* Routledge.

36. Claes, L., & Muehlenkamp, J. J. (2016). *Non-suicidal self-injury in eating disorders.* Springer-Verlag Berlin An.

37. Nock, M. K., Joiner, T. E., Jr., Gordon, K. H., Lloyd-Richardson, E., & Prinstein, M. J. (2006). Non-suicidal self-injury among adolescents: Diagnostic correlates and relation to suicide attempts. *Psychiatry Research, 144*(1), 65–72.

38. Peebles, R., Wilson, J. L., & Lock, J. D. (2011). Self-injury in adolescents with eating disorders: Correlates and provider bias. *Journal of Adolescent Health, 48*(3), 310–313.

39. Weierich, M. R., & Nock, M. K. (2008). Posttraumatic stress symptoms mediate the relation between childhood sexual abuse and nonsuicidal self-injury. *Journal of Consulting and Clinical Psychology, 76*(1), 39.

40. Cavanaugh, R. M. (2002). Self-mutilation as a manifestation of sexual abuse in adolescent girls. *Journal of Pediatric and Adolescent Gynecology, 15*(2), 97–100.

41. Noll, J. G., Horowitz, L. A., Bonanno, G. A., Trickett, P. K., & Putnam, F. W. (2003). Revictimization and self-harm in females who experienced childhood sexual abuse: Results from a prospective study. *Journal of Interpersonal Violence, 18*(12), 1452–1471.

42. Wonderlich, S., Donaldson, M. A., Carson, D. K., Staton, D., Gertz, L., Leach, L. R., & Johnson, M. (1996). Eating disturbance and incest. *Journal of Interpersonal Violence, 11*(2), 195–207.

43. Van der Kolk, B. A., Perry, J. C., & Herman, J. L. (1991). Childhood origins of self-destructive behavior. *American Journal of Psychiatry, 148*(12), 1665–1671.

44. Stone, M. H. (1987). A psychodynamic approach: Some thoughts on the dynamics and therapy of self-mutilating borderline patients. *Journal of Personality Disorders, 1*(4), 347–349.

45. Klonsky, E. D., & Moyer, A. (2008). Childhood sexual abuse and non-suicidal self-injury: Meta-analysis. *British Journal of Psychiatry, 192*(3), 166–170.

46. Andover, M. S. (2014). Non-suicidal self-injury disorder in a community sample of adults. *Psychiatry Research, 219*(2), 305–310.

47. Favazza, A. R., & Rosenthal, R. J. (1993). Diagnostic issues in self-mutilation. *Psychiatric Services, 44*(2), 134–140.

48. Muehlenkamp, J. J. (2005). Self-injurious behavior as a separate clinical syndrome. *American Journal of Orthopsychiatry, 75*(2), 324–333.

49. Selby, E. A., Bender, T. W., Gordon, K. H., Nock, M. K., & Joiner, T. E., Jr. (2012). Non-suicidal self-injury (NSSI) disorder: A preliminary study. *Personality Disorders: Theory, Research, and Treatment, 3*(2), 167.

50. Zetterqvist, M., Lundh, L. G., Dahlström, Ö., & Svedin, C. G. (2013). Prevalence and function of non-suicidal self-injury (NSSI) in a community sample of adolescents, using suggested DSM-5 criteria for a potential NSSI disorder. *Journal of Abnormal Child Psychology, 41*(5), 759–773.

51. American Psychiatric Association. (2013). *Diagnostic and statistical manual of mental disorders: DSM-5*. American Psychiatric Association.

52. Ammerman, B. A., Jacobucci, R., Kleiman, E. M., Muehlenkamp, J. J., & McCloskey, M. S. (2017). Development and validation of empirically derived frequency criteria for NSSI disorder using exploratory data mining. *Psychological Assessment, 29*(2), 221.

53. Glenn, C. R., & Klonsky, E. D. (2013). Nonsuicidal self-injury disorder: An empirical investigation in adolescent psychiatric patients. *Journal of Clinical Child and Adolescent Psychology, 42*(4), 496–507.

54. Muehlenkamp, J. J., Brausch, A. M., & Washburn, J. J. (2017). How much is enough? Examining frequency criteria for NSSI disorder in adolescent inpatients. *Journal of Consulting and Clinical Psychology, 85*(6), 611.

55. Selby, E. A., Kranzler, A., Fehling, K. B., & Panza, E. (2015). Nonsuicidal self-injury disorder: The path to diagnostic validity and final obstacles. *Clinical Psychology Review, 38*, 79–91.

56. Kiekens, G., Hasking, P., Claes, L., Mortier, P., Auerbach, R. P., Boyes, M., . . . Bruffaerts, R. (2018). The DSM-5 nonsuicidal self-injury disorder among incoming college students: Prevalence and associations with 12-month mental disorders and suicidal thoughts and behaviors. *Depression and Anxiety, 35*(7), 629–637.

57. Brausch, A. M., Muehlenkamp, J. J., & Washburn, J. J. (2016). Nonsuicidal self-injury disorder: Does Criterion B add diagnostic utility? *Psychiatry Research, 244*, 179–184.

58. Lewis, S. P., Bryant, L. A., Schaefer, B. M., & Grunberg, P. H. (2017). In their own words: Perspectives on nonsuicidal self-injury disorder among those with lived experience. *Journal of Nervous and Mental Disease, 205*(10), 771–779.

59. Staniland, L., Hasking, P., Boyes, M., & Lewis, S. (2021). Stigma and nonsuicidal self-injury: Application of a conceptual framework. *Stigma and Health, 6*(3), 312.

60. Heath, N. L., Toste, J. R., Sornberger, M. J., & Wagner, C. (2011). Teachers' perceptions of non-suicidal self-injury in the schools. *School Mental Health, 3*(1), 35–43.

61. Lewis, S. P., Mahdy, J. C., Michal, N. J., & Arbuthnott, A. E. (2014). Googling self-injury: The state of health information obtained through online searches for self-injury. *JAMA Pediatrics, 168*(5), 443–449.

62. Klonsky, E. D. (2007). The functions of deliberate self-injury: A review of the evidence. *Clinical Psychology Review, 27*(2), 226–239.

63. Taylor, P. J., Jomar, K., Dhingra, K., Forrester, R., Shahmalak, U., & Dickson, J. M. (2018). A meta-analysis of the prevalence of different functions of non-suicidal self-injury. *Journal of Affective Disorders, 227*, 759–769.

64. Klonsky, E. D., & Glenn, C. R. (2009). Assessing the functions of non-suicidal self-injury: Psychometric properties of the Inventory of Statements About Self-injury (ISAS). *Journal of Psychopathology and Behavioral Assessment, 31*(3), 215–219.

65. Nock, M. K., & Prinstein, M. J. (2004). A functional approach to the assessment of self-mutilative behavior. *Journal of Consulting and Clinical Psychology, 72*(5), 885.

66. Nock, M. K., & Prinstein, M. J. (2005). Contextual features and behavioral functions of self-mutilation among adolescents. *Journal of Abnormal Psychology, 114*(1), 140.

67. Bresin, K., & Gordon, K. H. (2013). Changes in negative affect following pain (vs. nonpainful) stimulation in individuals with and without a history of nonsuicidal self-injury. *Personality Disorders: Theory, Research, and Treatment, 4*(1), 62.

68. Bresin, K., Gordon, K. H., Bender, T. W., Gordon, L. J., & Joiner, T. E. (2010). No pain, no change: Reductions in prior negative affect following physical pain. *Motivation and Emotion, 34*(3), 280–287.

69. Franklin, J. C., Hessel, E. T., Aaron, R. V., Arthur, M. S., Heilbron, N., & Prinstein, M. J. (2010). The functions of nonsuicidal self-injury: Support for cognitive-affective regulation and opponent processes from a novel psychophysiological paradigm. *Journal of Abnormal Psychology, 119*(4), 850.

70. Fox, K. R., O'Sullivan, I. M., Wang, S. B., & Hooley, J. M. (2019). Self-criticism impacts emotional responses to pain. *Behavior Therapy, 50*(2), 410–420.

71. Fox, K. R., Ribeiro, J. D., Kleiman, E. M., Hooley, J. M., Nock, M. K., & Franklin, J. C. (2018). Affect toward the self and self-injury stimuli as potential risk factors for nonsuicidal self-injury. *Psychiatry Research, 260*, 279–285.

72. Zelkowitz, R. L., & Cole, D. A. (2019). Self-criticism as a transdiagnostic process in nonsuicidal self-injury and disordered eating: Systematic review and meta-analysis. *Suicide and Life-Threatening Behavior, 49*(1), 310–327.

73. Burke, T. A., Olino, T. M., & Alloy, L. B. (2017). Initial psychometric validation of the non-suicidal self-injury scar cognition scale. *Journal of Psychopathology and Behavioral Assessment, 39*(3), 546–562.

74. Burke, T. A., Piccirillo, M. L., Moore-Berg, S. L., Alloy, L. B., & Heimberg, R. G. (2019). The stigmatization of nonsuicidal self-injury. *Journal of Clinical Psychology, 75*(3), 481–498.

75. Lewis, S. P., & Mehrabkhani, S. (2016). Every scar tells a story: Insight into people's self-injury scar experiences. *Counselling Psychology Quarterly, 29*(3), 296–310.

76. Lewis, S. P. (2016). The overlooked role of self-injury scars: Commentary and suggestions for clinical practice. *Journal of Nervous and Mental Disease, 204*(1), 33–35.

77. Lewis, S. P., & Hasking, P. A. (2020). Rethinking self-injury recovery: A commentary and conceptual reframing. *BJPsych Bulletin, 44*(2), 44–46.

78. Lewis, S. P., & Hasking, P. A. (2021). Self-injury recovery: A person-centered framework. *Journal of Clinical Psychology, 77*(4), 884–895.

79. Lewis, S. P., & Hasking, P. (2019). Putting the "self" in self-injury research: Inclusion of people with lived experience in the research process. *Psychiatric Services, 70*(11), 1058–1060.

80. Lewis, S. P., & Hasking, P. A. (2021). Understanding self-injury: A person-centered approach. *Psychiatric Services, 72*(6), 721–723.

Chapter 2

1. National Institute for Health and Care Excellence (NICE). (2013). *Self-harm: Quality standard (QS34).* NICE; UK.

2. International Society for the Study of Self-Injury. (2018, May). What is self-injury? Retrieved from: https://itriples.org/category/about-self-injury/

3. Kapur, N., Cooper, J., O'Connor, R., & Hawton, K. (2013). Non-suicidal self-injury v. attempted suicide: New diagnosis or false dichotomy. *British Journal of Psychology, 202,* 326–328.

4. Klonsky, E. D., May, A. M., & Glenn, C. R. (2013). The relationship between nonsuicidal self-injury and attempted suicide: Converging evidence from four samples. *Journal of Abnormal Psychology, 122,* 231–237.

5. Hamza, C. A., Stewart, S. L., & Willoughby, T. (2012). Examining the link between nonsuicidal self-injury and suicidal behaviour: A review of the literature and an integrated model. *Clinical Psychology Review, 32,* 482–495.

6. Benjet, C., González-Herrera, I., Castro-Silva, E., Méndez, E., Borges, G., Casanova, L., & Medina-Mora, M. E. (2017). Non-suicidal self-injury in Mexican young adults: Prevalence, associations with suicidal behavior and psychiatric disorders, and DSM-5 proposed diagnostic criteria. *Journal of Affective Disorders, 215,* 1–8.

7. Martin, G., Swannell, S., Harrison, J., Hazell, P., & Taylor, A., 2010. *The Australian National Epidemiological Study of Self-Injury (ANESSI).* Centre for Suicide Prevention Studies, Discipline of Psychiatry. University of Queensland. Brisbane, Australia.

8. Whitlock, J., Muehlenkamp, J., Eckenrode, J., Purington, A., Baral Abrams, G., Barreira, P., & Kress, V. (2013). Nonsuicidal self-injury as a gateway to suicide in young adults. *Journal of Adolescent Health, 52,* 486–492.

9. Joiner, T. E. (2005). *Why people die by suicide.* Harvard University Press.

10. Van Orden, K. A., Witte, T. K., Cukrowicz, K. C., Braithwaite, S., Selby, E. A., & Joiner, T. E. (2010). The interpersonal theory of suicide. *Psychological Review, 117,* 575–600.

11. Koening, J., Thayer, J. F., & Kaess, M. (2016). A meta-analysis on pain sensitivity in self-injury. *Psychological Medicine, 46,* 1597–1612.

12. Gordon, K. H., Selby, E. A., Anestis, M. D., Bender, T. W., Witte, T. K., Braithwaite, S., Van Orden, K. A., Bresin, K., & Joiner, T. E. (2010). The reinforcing properties of repeated deliberate self-harm. *Archives of Suicide Research, 14,* 329–341.

13. St Germain, S. A., & Hooley, J. M. (2013). Aberrant pain perception in direct and indirect non-suicidal self-injury: An empirical test of Joiner's interpersonal theory. *Comprehensive Psychiatry, 54,* 694–701.

14. Law, K. C., Khazem, L. R., Jin, H. M., & Anestis, M. D. (2017). Non-social self-injury and frequency of suicide attempts: The role of pain persistence. *Journal of Affective Disorders, 209,* 254–261.

15. Heffer, T., & Willoughby, T. (2018). The role of emotion dysregulation: A longitudinal investigation of the interpersonal theory of suicide. *Psychiatry Research, 260*, 379–383.

16. Muehlenkamp, J. J., Hilt, L. M., Ehlinger, P. P., & McMillan, T. (2015). Nonsuicidal self-injury in sexual minority college students: A test of theoretical integration. *Child and Adolescent Psychiatry and Mental Health, 9*, 16.

17. Chu, C., Rogers, M. L., & Joiner, T. E. (2016). Cross-sectional and temporal associations between non-suicidal self-injury and suicidal ideation in young adults: The explanatory roles of thwarted belongingness and perceive burdensomeness. *Psychiatry Research, 246*, 573–580.

18. Chu, C., Hom, M. A., Stanley, I. H., Gai, A. R., Nock, M. K., Gutierrez, P. M., & Joiner, T. E. (2018). Non-suicidal self-injury and suicidal thoughts and behaviours: A study of the explanatory roles of the interpersonal theory variables among military service members and veterans. *Journal of Consulting and Clinical Psychology, 86*, 56–68.

19. Barzilay, S., Feldman, D., Snir, A., Apter, A., Carli, V., Hoven, C. W., Wasserman, C., Sarchiapone, M., & Wasserman, D. (2015). The interpersonal theory of suicide and adolescent suicidal behaviour. *Journal of Affective Disorders, 183*, 68–74.

20. Christensen, H., Batterhham, P. J., Soubelet, A., & MacKinnon, A. J. (2013). A test of the interpersonal theory of suicide in a large community-based cohort. *Journal of Affective Disorders, 144*, 225–234.

21. Kiekens, G., Hasking, P., Claes, L., Boyes, M., Mortier, P., Auerbach, R. P., Cuijpers, P., Demyttenaere, K., Green, J. G., Kessler, R. C., Nock, M. K., & Bruffaerts, R. (2018). The associations between non-suicidal self-injury and first onset suicidal thoughts and behaviors. *Journal of Affective Disorders, 239*, 171–179.

22. Kiekens, G., Hasking, P., Claes, L., Mortier, P., Auerbach, R., Boyes, M., Cuijpers, P., Demyttenaere, K., Green, J., Kessler, R., Nock, M., & Bruffaerts, R. (2018). The DSM-5 non-suicidal self-injury disorder among college freshman: Prevalence and associations with mental disorders and suicidal thoughts and behaviours. *Depression and Anxiety, 35*, 629–637.

23. Victor, S. E., Styer, D., & Washburn, J. J. (2015). Characteristics of nonsuicidal self-injury associated with suicidal ideation: Evidence from a clinical sample of youth. *Child and Adolescent Psychiatry and Mental Health, 9*(1), 1–8.

24. Franklin, J. C., Ribeiro, J. D., Fox, K. R., Bentley, K. H., Kleiman, E. M., Huang, X., Musacchio, K. M., Jaroszewski, A. C., Chang, B. P., & Nock, M. K. (2017). Risk factors for suicidal thoughts and behaviours: A meta-analysis of 50 years of research. *Psychological Bulletin, 143*, 187–232.

25. Ribeiro, J. D., Franklin, J. C., Fox, K. R., Bentley, K. H., Kleiman, E. M., Chang, B. P., & Nock, M. K. (2016). Self-injurious thoughts and behaviours as risk factors for future suicide ideation, attempts, and death: A meta-analysis of longitudinal studies. *Psychological Medicine, 46*, 225–236.

26. Kettlewell, C. (1999). *Skin game: A memoir*. St Martin's Griffin.

27. Hunter Institute of Mental Health. (2012). *Summary of the literature for discussing suicide*. Newcastle, Australia.

28. Beaton, S., Forster, P., & Maple. M. (2013). Suicide and language: Why we shouldn't use the "C" word. *InPsych, February, 35*(1), 30–31.

29. Stanley, B., & Brown, G. K. (2012). A brief intervention to mitigate suicide risk. *Cognitive and Behavioral Practice, 19*, 256–264.

30. Kelada, L., Hasking, P., Melvin, G., Whitlock, J., & Baetens, I. (2018). "I do want to stop, at least I think I do": An international comparison of recovery from nonsuicidal self-injury among young people. *Journal of Adolescent Research, 33*, 416–441.

31. Gray, N., Hasking, P., & Boyes, M. (2021). The impact of ambivalence on recovery from non-suicidal self-injury: Considerations for health professionals. *Journal of Public Mental Health, 20*(4), 251–258.

Chapter 3

1. Chapman, A. L., Gratz, K. L., & Brown, M. Z. (2006). Solving the puzzle of deliberate self-harm: The experiential avoidance model. *Behaviour, Research, and Therapy, 44*, 371–394.

2. Nock, M. K. (2009). Why do people hurt themselves? New insights into the nature and functions of self-injury. *Current Directions in Psychological Science, 18*, 78–83.

3. Selby, E. A., & Joiner, T. E. (2009). Cascades of emotion: The emergence of borderline personality disorder from emotional and behavioural dysregulation. *Review of General Psychology, 13*, 219–229.

4. Hasking, P., Whitlock, J., Voon, D., & Rose, A. (2017). A cognitive-emotional model of NSSI: Using emotion regulation and cognitive processes to explain why people self-injure. *Cognition and Emotion, 31*, 1543–1556.

5. Bandura, A. (1986). *Social foundations of thought and action: A social cognitive theory*. Prentice-Hall.

6. Dawkins, J., Hasking, P., & Boyes, M. (2021). Thoughts and beliefs about nonsuicidal self-injury: An application of social cognitive theory. *Journal of American College Health, 69*, 428–434.

7. Hooley, J. M., & Franklin, J. C. (2018). Why do people hurt themselves? A new conceptual model of nonsuicidal self-injury. *Clinical Psychological Science, 6, 428–451.*

8. Hasking, P., Lewis, S. P., & Boyes, M. (2021). The language of self-injury: A data-informed commentary. *Journal of Nervous and Mental Disease, 209*, 233–236.

9. Hasking, P., & Boyes, M. (2018). Cutting words: A commentary on language and stigma in the context of non-suicidal self-injury. *Journal of Nervous and Mental Disease, 206*, 829–833.

10. Hasking, P., Lewis, S. P., & Boyes, M. (2019). When language is maladaptive: Recommendations for discussing self-injury. *Journal of Public Mental Health, 18*, 148–152.

11. Lewis, S. P., & Hasking, P. A. (2020). Rethinking self-injury recovery: A commentary and conceptual reframing. *BJPsych Bulletin, 44*(2), 44–46.

12. Lewis, S. P., & Hasking, P. (2021). Self-injury recovery: A person-centred framework. *Journal of Clinical Psychology, 77*, 884–895.

13. Lewis, S. P., & Hasking, P. (2020). Putting the self in self-injury research: Inclusion of people with lived experience in research. *Psychiatric Services, 70*, 1058–1060.

14. Lewis, S. P., & Hasking, P. (2021). Understanding self-injury: A person-centred approach. *Psychiatric Services, 72*, 721–723.

15. Schutte, N. S., & Malouff, J. M. (2019). The impact of signature character strengths interventions: A meta-analysis. *Journal of Happiness Studies, 20*, 1179–1196.

16. Padesky, C. A., & Mooney, K. A. (2012). Strengths-based cognitive-behavioural therapy: A four-step model to build resilience. *Clinical Psychology and Psychotherapy, 19*, 283–290.

17. Victor, P. P., Teisman, T., & Willutzki, U. (2017). A pilot evaluation of a strengths-based CBT intervention module with college students. *Behavioural and Cognitive Psychotherapy, 45*, 427–431.

18. Peterson, C., & Seligman, M. E. P. (2004). *Character strengths and virtues: A classification and handbook.* American Psychological Association.

19. McAllister, M., Hasking, P. A., Estefan, A., McClenaghan, K., & Lowe, J. (2010). A strengths-based group program on self-harm: A feasibility study. *Journal of School Nursing, 26*, 289–300.

20. McAllister, M., Knight, B., Hasking, P., Withyman, C., & Dawkins, J. (2018). Building resilience in regional youth: Impacts of a universal mental health promotion program. *International Journal of Mental Health Nursing, 27*, 1044–1054.

21. McAllister, M., Knight, B. A., Handley, C., Dawkins, J., Sargent, L., Walters, V., & Hasking, P. (2019). Evaluation of a professional development experience designed to equip school support staff with skills to facilitate youth mental health promotion. *Contemporary Nurse, 55*, 408–420.

22. de Wit, M., Cooper, C., Reginster, J., on behalf of the WHO-ESCO Working Group. (2019). Practical guidance for patient-centred health research. *Lancet, 393*, 1095–1096.

23. Gluyas, H. (2015). Patient-centred care: Improving healthcare outcomes. *Nursing Standard, 30*, 50–57.

24. Santana, M. J., Manalili, K., Jolley, R. J., Zelinsky, S., Quan, H., & Lu, M. (2018). How to practice person-centred care: A conceptual framework. *Health Expectations, 21*, 429–440.

25. Kuipers, S. J., Cramm, J. M., & Nieboer, A. P. (2019). The importance of patient-centred care and co-creation of care for satisfaction with care and physical and social wellbeing of patients with multi-morbidity in the primary care setting. *BMC Health Services Research, 19*, 13.

26. Gray, N., Hasking, P., & Boyes, M. E. (2021). The impact of ambivalence on recovery from non-suicidal self-injury: Considerations for health professionals. *Journal of Public Mental Health, 20*(4), 251–258.

27. Lloyd-Richardson, E., Hasking, P., Lewis, S., Hamza, C., McAllister, M., Baetens, I., & Muehlenkamp, J. (2020). Understanding non-suicidal self-injury and the importance of respectful curiosity in supporting youth who engage in self-injury. *NASN School Nurse, 35*, 92–98.

28. Hasking, P. A., Bloom, E., Lewis, S. P., & Baetens, I. (2020). Developing a policy, and professional development for school staff, to address and respond to nonsuicidal self-injury in schools. *International Perspectives in Psychology: Research, Practice, Consultation, 9*, 176–179.

29. Lewis, S. P., Heath, N. L., Hasking, P. A., Hamza, C., Bloom, E., Lloyd-Richardson, E., & Whitlock, J. (2020). Advocacy for improved response to self-injury in schools: A call to action for school psychologists. *Psychological Services, 17*, 86–92.

Chapter 4

1. Burke, T. A., Piccirillo, M. L., Moore-Berg, S. L., Alloy, L. B., & Heimberg, R. G. (2019). The stigmatization of nonsuicidal self-injury. *Journal of Clinical Psychology*, *75*(3), 481–498.

2. Long, M. (2018). "We're not monsters . . . we're just really sad sometimes": Hidden self-injury, stigma and help-seeking. *Health Sociology Review*, *27*(1), 89–103.

3. Piccirillo, M. L., Burke, T. A., Moore-Berg, S. L., Alloy, L. B., & Heimberg, R. G. (2020). Self-stigma toward nonsuicidal self-injury: An examination of implicit and explicit attitudes. *Suicide and Life-Threatening Behavior*, *50*(5), 1007–1024.

4. Staniland, L., Hasking, P., Boyes, M., & Lewis, S. (2021). Stigma and nonsuicidal self-injury: Application of a conceptual framework. *Stigma and Health*, *6*(3), 312.

5. Corrigan, P. W., & Rao, D. (2012). On the self-stigma of mental illness: Stages, disclosure, and strategies for change. *Canadian Journal of Psychiatry*, *57*(8), 464–469.

6. Corrigan, P. W., & Watson, A. C. (2002). The paradox of self-stigma and mental illness. *Clinical Psychology: Science and Practice*, *9*(1), 35.

7. Link, B. G., Yang, L. H., Phelan, J. C., & Collins, P. Y. (2004). Measuring mental illness stigma. *Schizophrenia Bulletin*, *30*(3), 511–541.

8. Lewis, S. P., Mahdy, J. C., Michal, N. J., & Arbuthnott, A. E. (2014). Googling self-injury: The state of health information obtained through online searches for self-injury. *JAMA Pediatrics*, *168*(5), 443–449.

9. Lloyd, B., Blazely, A., & Phillips, L. (2018). Stigma towards individuals who self harm: Impact of gender and disclosure. *Journal of Public Mental Health*, *17*(4), 184–194.

10. Lund, E. M., Schultz, J. C., Nadorff, M. R., Thomas, K. B., Chowdhury, D., & Galbraith, K. (2018). Experiences with and knowledge of non-suicidal self-injury in vocational rehabilitation support staff. *Journal of Applied Rehabilitation Counseling*, *49*(1), 32–39.

11. Sandy, P. T., & Shaw, D. G. (2012). Attitudes of mental health nurses to self-harm in secure forensic settings: A multi-method phenomenological investigation. *Journal of Medicine and Medical Science Research*, *1*(4), 63–75.

12. Hughes, N. D., Locock, L., Simkin, S., Stewart, A., Ferrey, A. E., Gunnell, D., . . . Hawton, K. (2017). Making sense of an unknown terrain: How parents understand self-harm in young people. *Qualitative Health Research*, *27*(2), 215–225.

13. Oldershaw, A., Richards, C., Simic, M., & Schmidt, U. (2008). Parents' perspectives on adolescent self-harm: Qualitative study. *British Journal of Psychiatry*, *193*(2), 140–144.

14. Mitten, N., Preyde, M., Lewis, S., Vanderkooy, J., & Heintzman, J. (2016). The perceptions of adolescents who self-harm on stigma and care following inpatient psychiatric treatment. *Social Work in Mental Health*, *14*(1), 1–21.

15. Chandler, A. (2014). Narrating the self-injured body. *Medical Humanities*, *40*(2), 111–116.

16. Scambler, G. (1998). Stigma and disease: Changing paradigms. *Lancet*, *352*(9133), 1054–1055.

17. Quinn, D. M., & Chaudoir, S. R. (2009). Living with a concealable stigmatized identity: The impact of anticipated stigma, centrality, salience, and cultural stigma on psychological distress and health. *Journal of Personality and Social Psychology*, *97*(4), 634.

18. Hasking, P., Staniland, L., Boyes, M., & Lewis, S.P. (in review). *Adding insult to injury: The accumulation of stigmatizing language on individuals with lived experience of self-injury.*

19. Gibb, S. J., Beautrais, A. L., & Surgenor, L. J. (2010). Health-care staff attitudes towards self-harm patients. *Australian and New Zealand Journal of Psychiatry, 44*(8), 713–720.

20. Karman, P., Kool, N., Poslawsky, I. E., & van Meijel, B. (2015). Nurses' attitudes towards self-harm: A literature review. *Journal of Psychiatric and Mental Health Nursing, 22*(1), 65–75.

21. Saunders, K. E., Hawton, K., Fortune, S., & Farrell, S. (2012). Attitudes and knowledge of clinical staff regarding people who self-harm: A systematic review. *Journal of Affective Disorders, 139*(3), 205–216.

22. Berger, E., Reupert, A., & Hasking, P. (2015). Pre-service and in-service teachers' knowledge, attitudes and confidence towards self-injury among pupils. *Journal of Education for Teaching, 41*(1), 37–51.

23. Heath, N. L., Toste, J. R., Sornberger, M. J., & Wagner, C. (2011). Teachers' perceptions of non-suicidal self-injury in the schools. *School Mental Health, 3*(1), 35–43.

24. Rosenrot, S. A., & Lewis, S. P. (2020). Barriers and responses to the disclosure of non-suicidal self-injury: A thematic analysis. *Counselling Psychology Quarterly, 33*(2), 121–141.

25. Mahtani, S., Melvin, G. A., & Hasking, P. (2018). Shame proneness, shame coping, and functions of nonsuicidal self-injury (NSSI) among emerging adults: A developmental analysis. *Emerging Adulthood, 6*(3), 159–171.

26. Corrigan, P. (2004). How stigma interferes with mental health care. *American Psychologist, 59*(7), 614.

27. Jackson-Best, F., & Edwards, N. (2018). Stigma and intersectionality: A systematic review of systematic reviews across HIV/AIDS, mental illness, and physical disability. *BMC Public Health, 18*(1), 1–19.

28. Jones, E. E., Farina, A., Hastorf, A. H., Markus, H., Miller, D. T., & Scott, R. A. (1984). *Social stigma: The psychology of marked relationships.* W. H. Freeman and Company.

29. Weiner, B., Perry, R. P., & Magnusson, J. (1988). An attributional analysis of reactions to stigmas. *Journal of Personality and Social Psychology, 55*(5), 738.

30. Burke, T. A., Ammerman, B. A., Hamilton, J. L., & Alloy, L. B. (2017). Impact of non-suicidal self-injury scale: Initial psychometric validation. *Cognitive Therapy and Research, 41*(1), 130–142.

31. Weiner, B. (1995). *Judgments of responsibility: A foundation for a theory of social conduct.* Guilford.

32. Lewis, S. P., & Hasking, P. A. (2020). Rethinking self-injury recovery: A commentary and conceptual reframing. *BJPsych Bulletin, 44*(2), 44–46.

33. Lewis, S. P., & Hasking, P. A. (2021). Self-injury recovery: A person-centered framework. *Journal of Clinical Psychology, 77*(4), 884–895.

34. Lewis, S. P. (2016). The overlooked role of self-injury scars: Commentary and suggestions for clinical practice. *Journal of Nervous and Mental Disease, 204*(1), 33–35.

35. McAllister, M., Creedy, D., Moyle, W., & Farrugia, C. (2002). Nurses' attitudes towards clients who self-harm. *Journal of Advanced Nursing, 40*(5), 578–586.

36. Rissanen, M. L., Kylmä, J., & Laukkanen, E. (2009). Descriptions of help by Finnish adolescents who self-mutilate. *Journal of Child and Adolescent Psychiatric Nursing, 22,* 7–15.

37. Lewis, S. P., & Mehrabkhani, S. (2016). Every scar tells a story: Insight into people's self-injury scar experiences. *Counselling Psychology Quarterly, 29,* 296–310.

38. Frankham, E. (2019). A modified framework for identifying stigma: News coverage of persons with mental illness killed by police. *Stigma and Health, 4,* 62–71.

39. Stuart, H. (2006). Media portrayal of mental illness and its treatments. *CNS drugs, 20*(2), 99–106.

40. Corrigan, P. W., Watson, A. C., Gracia, G., Slopen, N., Rasinski, K., & Hall, L. L. (2005). Newspaper stories as measures of structural stigma. *Psychiatric Services, 56*(5), 551–556.

41. Lewis, S. P., & Hasking, P. (2019). Putting the "self" in self-injury research: Inclusion of people with lived experience in the research process. *Psychiatric Services, 70*(11), 1058–1060.

42. Lewis, S.P., Heath, N.L., & Whitley, R. (in press). Addressing self-injury stigma: The promise of innovative digital and video action-research methods. *Canadian Journal of Community Mental Health.*

43. Nielsen, E., & Townsend, E. (2018). Public perceptions of self-harm: A test of an attribution model of public discrimination. *Stigma and Health, 3,* 204–218.

44. Day, E. N., Edgren, K., & Eshleman, A. (2007). Measuring stigma toward mental illness: Development and application of the mental illness stigma scale 1. *Journal of Applied Social Psychology, 37*(10), 2191–2219.

45. King, M., Dinos, S., Shaw, J., Watson, R., Stevens, S., Passetti, F., & Serfaty, M. (2007). The Stigma Scale: Development of a standardised measure of the stigma of mental illness. *British Journal of Psychiatry, 190*(3), 248–254.

46. Staniland, L., Hasking, P., Boyes, M., & Lewis, S.P. (in preparation). Development and Validation of the Self-Injury Stigma Questionnaire.

47. Griffiths, K. M., Carron-Arthur, B., Parsons, A., & Reid, R. (2014). Effectiveness of programs for reducing the stigma associated with mental disorders: A meta-analysis of randomized controlled trials. *World Psychiatry, 13*(2), 161–175.

48. Mehta, N., Clement, S., Marcus, E., Stona, A. C., Bezborodovs, N., Evans-Lacko, S., . . . Thornicroft, G. (2015). Evidence for effective interventions to reduce mental health-related stigma and discrimination in the medium and long term: Systematic review. *British Journal of Psychiatry, 207*(5), 377–384.

49. Thornicroft, G., Mehta, N., Clement, S., Evans-Lacko, S., Doherty, M., Rose, D., . . . Henderson, C. (2016). Evidence for effective interventions to reduce mental-health-related stigma and discrimination. *Lancet, 387*(10023), 1123–1132.

Chapter 5

1. Bo, C. (2015). Social constructivism of language and meaning. *Croatian Journal of Philosophy, 43,* 87–113.

2. Slovenko, R. (2001). The stigma of psychiatric discourse. *Journal of Psychiatry and Law, 29,* 5–29.

3. Ross, A. M., Morgan, A. J., Jorm, A. F., & Reavley, N. J. (2019). A systematic review of the impact of media reports of severe mental illness on stigma and discrimination, and interventions that aim to mitigate any adverse impact. *Social Psychiatry and Psychiatric Epidemiology, 54*, 11–31.

4. Black, M., & Downie, J. (2010). Watch your language: A review of the use of stigmatizing language by Canadian judges. *Journal of Ethics in Mental Health, 5*, 1–8.

5. Staniland, L., Hasking, P., Boyes, M., & Lewis, S. (2021). Stigma and nonsuicidal self-injury: Application of a conceptual framework. *Stigma and Health, 6*, 312–323.

6. Hogg, M. A., Abrams, D., & Brewer, M. B. (2017). Social identity: The role of self in group processes and intergroup relations. *Group Processes an Intergroup Relations, 20*, 570–581.

7. Festinger L. (1954). A theory of social comparison processes. *Human Relations, 7*, 117–140.

8. Burgers, C., Beukeboom, C. J., Kelder, M., & Peeters, M. M. E. (2015). How sports fans forge intergroup competition though language: The case of verbal irony. *Communication Research, 41*, 435–457.

9. Maas, A., Ceccarelli, R., & Rudin, S. (1996). Linguistic intergroup bias: Evidence for in-group-protective motivation. *Journal of Personality and Asocial Psychology, 71*, 512–526.

10. Porter, S.C, Rheinschmidt-Same, M., & Richeson, J. A. (2015). Inferring identity from language: Linguistic intergroup bias informs social categorisation. *Psychological Science, 27*, 1–9.

11. Fausey, C. M., & Boroditsky, L. (2010). Subtle linguistic cues influence perceived blame and financial liability. *Psychological Bulletin and Review, 17*, 644–650.

12. Krauss, R. M., & Chiu, C. (1997). Language and social behavior. In D. Gilbert, S. Fiske, & G. Lindsey (Eds.), *Handbook of social psychology* (Vol. 2, pp. 41–88). McGraw-Hill.

13. Tsfati, Y., & Ariely, G. (2014). Individual and contextual correlates of trust in media across 44 countries. *Communication Research, 41*, 760–782.

14. American Psychiatric Association. (2013). *Diagnostic and statistical manual of mental disorders* (5th ed.). Author.

15. Hasking, P., & Boyes, M. (2018). Cutting words: A commentary on language and stigma in the context of non-suicidal self-injury. *Journal of Nervous and Mental Disease, 206*, 829–833.

16. Hasking, P., Heath, N. L., Kaess, M., Lewis, S. P., Plener, P. L., Walsh, B. W., Whitlock, J., & Wilson, M. S. (2016). Position paper for guiding response to non-suicidal self-injury in schools. *School Psychology International, 37*, 644–663.

17. Wester, K. L., Morris, C. W., & Williams, B. (2018). Nonsuicidal self-injury in the schools: A tiered prevention approach for reducing social contagion. *Professional School Counseling, 21*, 142–151.

18. Gratz, K. L., & Chapman, A. L. (2009). *Freedom from self-harm: Overcoming self-injury with skills from DBT and other treatments*. New Harbinger Publications.

19. Recovery. (2020). *Oxford English Dictionary*. Available at: https://www.lexico.com/definition/recovery

20. Nixon, M. K., Cloutier, P. F., & Aggarwal. S. (2002). Affect regulation and addictive aspects of repetitive self-injury in hospitalized adolescents. *Journal of the American Academy of Child and Adolescent Psychiatry, 41*, 1333–1341.

21. Lewis, S. P., & Baker, T. G. (2011). The possible risks of self-injury web sites: A content analysis. *Archives of Suicide Research, 15*(4), 390–396.
22. Victor, S. E., Glenn, C. R., & Klonsky, E. D. (2012). Is non-suicidal self-injury an "addiction"? A comparison of craving in substance use and non-suicidal self-injury. *Psychiatry Research, 197,* 73–77.
23. Lewis, S. P., & Hasking, P. A. (2020). Rethinking self-injury recovery: A commentary and conceptual reframing. *BJPsych Bulletin, 44*(2), 44–46.
24. Lewis, S. P., & Hasking, P. (2021). Understanding self-injury: A person-centred approach. *Psychiatric Services, 72,* 721–723.
25. Hasking, P., Lewis, S. P., & Boyes, M. (2019). When language is maladaptive: Recommendations for discussing self-injury. *Journal of Public Mental Health, 18,* 148–152.
26. Lewis, S. P. (2017). I cut therefore I am? Avoiding labels in the context of self-injury. *Medical Humanities, 43,* 204.
27. Hasking, P., Lewis, S. P., & Boyes, M. (2021). The language of self-injury: A data-informed commentary. *Journal of Nervous and Mental Disease, 209,* 233–236.

Chapter 6

1. Hasking, P. A., Andrews, T., & Martin, G. (2013). The role of exposure to self-injury among peers in predicting later self-injury. *Journal of Youth and Adolescence, 42,* 1543–1556.
2. Prinstein, M. J., Heilbron, N., Guerry, J. D., Franklin, J. C., Rancourt, D., Simon, V., & Spirito, A. (2010). Peer influence and nonsuicidal self-injury: Longitudinal results in community and clinically-referred adolescent samples. *Journal of Abnormal Child Psychology, 38,* 669–682.
3. Schwartz-Mette, R. A., & Lawrence, H. R. (2019), Peer socialization of non-suicidal self-injury in adolescents' close friendships. *Journal of Abnormal Child Psychology, 47,* 1851–1862.
4. Hasking, P., & Rose, A. (2016). A preliminary application of social cognitive theory to nonsuicidal self-injury. *Journal of Youth and Adolescence, 45,* 1560–1574.
5. Heath, N. L., Ross, S., Toste, J. R., Charlebois, A., & Nedecheva, T. (2009). Retrospective analysis of social factors and nonsuicidal self-injury among young adults. *Canadian Journal of Behavioural Science, 41,* 180–186.
6. Muehlenkamp, J. J., Brausch, A., Quiqlry, K., & Whitlock, J. (2013). Interpersonal features and functions of nonsuicidal self-injury. *Suicide and Life-Threatening Behaviour, 43,* 67–80.
7. Claes, L., Houben, A., Vandereycken, W., Bijttebier, P., & Muehlenkamp, J. (2010). The association between non-suicidal self-injury, self-concept, and acquaintance with self-injurious peers in a sample of adolescents. *Journal of Adolescence, 33,* 775–778.
8. Brooks, A. (2015). Understanding the social functions of nonsuicidal self-injury in community adolescents. *Canadian Journal of Counselling and Psychotherapy, 49,* 296–314.
9. Jarvi, S., Jackson, B., Swenson, L., & Crawford, H. (2013). The impact of social contagion on non-suicidal self-injury: A review of the literature. *Archives of Suicide Research, 17,* 1–19.

10. Deliberto, T. L., & Nock, M. K. (2008). An exploratory study of correlates, onset, and offset of non-suicidal self-injury. *Archives of Suicide Research, 12*, 219–231.

11. You, J., Lin, M. P., & Leung, F. (2013). The best friend and friendship group influence on nonsuicidal self-injury. *Journal of Abnormal Child Psychology, 41*, 993–1004.

12. Zhu, L., Westers, N.J, Horton, S. E., King, J. D., Diederich, A., Stewart, S. M., & Kennard, B. D. (2016). Frequency of exposure to and engagement in nonsuicidal self-injury among inpatient adolescents. *Archives of Suicide Research, 20*, 580–590.

13. Stack, S. (2003). Media coverage a risk factor in suicide. *Journal of Epidemiology and Community Health, 57*, 238–240.

14. Pirkis, J., & Blood, R. W. (2001). *Suicide and the media: A critical review.* Canberra: Commonwealth Department of Health and Aged Care.

15. Lewis, S. P., Hasking, P. A., Staniland, L., Collaton, J., Boyes, M., & Bryce, L. (in revision). Self-injury in the news: A content analysis. *Media, Culture, and Society.*

16. Westers, N. J., Lewis, S. P., Whitlock, J., Schatten, H. T., Ammerman, B., Andover, M. S., & Lloyd-Richardson, E. E. (2021). Media guidelines for the responsible reporting and depicting of non-suicidal self-injury. *British Journal of Psychiatry, 219*(2), 415–418.

17. Nixon, M. K., Cloutier, P., & Jansson, S. M. (2008). Nonsuicidal self-injury in youth: A population-based survey. *Canadian Medical Association Journal, 178*, 306–312.

18. Bandura, A. (1977). *Social learning theory.* Prentice Hall.

19. Trewavas, C., Hasking, P. A., & McAllister, M. (2010). Representations of non-suicidal self-injury in motion pictures. *Archives of Suicide Research, 14*, 89–103.

20. Lewis, S. P., & Yeko, Y. (2016). A double-edged sword: A review of benefits and risks of online nonsuicidal self-injury activities. *Journal of Clinical Psychology, 72*, 249–262.

21. Lloyd-Richardson, E. E., Perrine, N., Dierker, L., & Kelly, M. L. (2007). Characteristics and functions of non-suicidal self-injury in a community sample of adolescents, *Psychological Medicine, 37*, 1183–1192.

22. Young, R., Sweeting, H., & West, P. (2006). Prevalence of deliberate self-harm and attempted suicide within contemporary Goth youth subculture: Longitudinal cohort study. *British Medical Journal, 332*, 1058–1061.

23. Young, R., Sproeber, N., Groschwitz, R., Priess, M., & Plener, P. L. (2014). Why alternative teenagers self-harm: Exploring the link between non-suicidal self-injury, attempted suicide and adolescent identity. *BMC Psychiatry, 14*, 137.

24. Klonsky, E. D., & Olino, T. M. (2008). Identifying clinically distinct subgroups of self-injurers among young adults: A latent class analysis. *Journal of Consulting and Clinical Psychology, 76*, 22–27.

25. Lindholm, T., Bjärehed, J., & Lundh, L. (2011). Functions of nonsuicidal self-injury among young women in residential care: A pilot study with the Swedish version of the Inventory of Statements About Self-Injury. *Cognitive Behaviour Therapy, 40*, 183–189.

26. Bajetan, K., Swenson, L. P., Jarvi, S. M., & Muehlenkamp, J. J. (2015). Perceptions of the functions of nonsuicidal self-injury in a college sample. *Crisis, 36*, 338–344.

27. Brausch, A. M., & Muehlenkamp, J. J. (2018). Perceived effectiveness of NSSI in achieving functions on severity and suicide risk. *Psychiatry Research, 265*, 144–150.

28. Bandura, A. (1986). *Social foundations of thought and action: A social cognitive theory*. Prentice-Hall.

29. Hasking, P., Whitlock, J., Voon, D., & Rose, A. (2017). A cognitive-emotional model of NSSI: Using emotion regulation and cognitive processes to explain why people self-injure. *Cognition and Emotion, 31*, 1543–1556.

30. Dawkins, J., Hasking, P., & Boyes, M. (2021). Thoughts and beliefs about nonsuicidal self-injury: An application of social cognitive theory. *Journal of American College Health, 69*, 428–434.

31. Dawkins, J., Hasking, P., & Boyes, M. (2019). Knowledge of parental nonsuicidal self-injury in young people who self-injure: The mediating role of outcome expectancies. *Journal of Family Studies, 27*(4), 479–490.

32. Wood, A., Trainor, G., Rothwell, J., Moore, A., & Harrington, R. (2001). Randomized controlled trial of group therapy for repeated deliberate self-harm in adolescents. *Journal of the American Academy of Child and Adolescent Psychiatry, 40*, 1246–1253.

33. Hazell, P. L., Martin, G., McGill, K., Kay, T., Wood, A., Trainor, G., & Harrington, R. (2009). Group therapy for repeated deliberate self-harm in adolescents: Failure of a replication of a randomised trial. *Journal of the American Academy of Child and Adolescent Psychiatry, 48*, 6662–670.

34. Green, J. M., Wood, A. J., Kerfoot, M. J., Trainor, G., Roberts, C., Rothwell, J., Woodham, A., Ayodeji, E., Barret, B., Byford, S., & Harrington, R. (2011). Group therapy for adolescents with repeated self-harm: Randomised controlled trial with economic evaluation. *British Medical Journal, 342*, d682.

35. Gratz, K. L., & Gunderson, J. G. (2006). Preliminary data on an acceptance-based emotion regulation group intervention for deliberate self-harm among women with borderline personality disorder. *Behavior Therapy, 37*, 25–35.

36. Gratz, K. L., Tull, M. T., & Levy, R. (2014). Randomised controlled trial and un-controlled 9-month follow-up of an adjunctive emotion regulation group therapy for deliberate self-harm among women with borderline personality disorder. *Psychological Medicine, 44*, 2099–2112.

37. Martin, S., Martin, G., Lequertier, B., Swannell, S., Follent, A., & Choe, F. (2012). Voice movement therapy: An evaluation of a group-based expressive arts therapy for nonsuicidal self-injury in young adults. *Music and Medicine, 5*, 31–38.

38. Rosen, P. M., & Walsh, B. W. (1989). Patterns of contagion in self-mutilation epidemics. *American Journal of Psychiatry, 146*, 656–658.

39. Taiminen, T. J., Kallio-Soukainen, K., Nokso-Koivisto, H., Kaljonen, A., & Helenius, H. (1998). Contagion of deliberate self-harm among adolescent inpatients. *Journal of the American Academy of Child and Adolescent Psychiatry, 37*, 211–217.

40. Cawthorpe, D., Somers, D., Wilkes, T., & Phil, M. (2003). Behavioural contagion reconsidered: Self-harm among adolescent psychiatry inpatients: A five-year study. *Canadian Child and Adolescent Psychiatry Review, 12*(4), 103–106.

41. Muelenkamp, J. J., Walsh, B. W., & McDade, M. (2010). Preventing non-suicidal self-injury in adolescents: The signs of self-injury program. *Journal of Youth and Adolescence, 39*, 306–314.

42. Robinson, J., Yuen, H. P., Martin, C., Hughes, A., Baksheev, G. N., Dodd, S., Bapat, S., Schwass, W., McGorry, P., & Yung, A. (2011). Does screening high school students for psychological distress, deliberate self-harm, or suicidal ideation cause distress—and is it acceptable? *Crisis, 32*, 254–263.

43. Albert, D., Cheing, J., & Steinberg, L. (2013). The teenage brain: Peer influences on adolescent decision making. *Current Directions in Psychological Science, 22,* 114–120.

44. Gould, M. S., Marrocco, F. A., Kleinman, M., Thomas, J. G., Mostkoff, K., Cote, J., & Davies, M. (2005). Evaluating iatrogenic effects of youth suicide screening programs: A randomized control trial. *Journal of the American Medical Association, 293,* 1635–1643.

45. Muehlenkamp, J. J., Swenson, L. P., Batejan, K. L., & Jarvi, S. (2014). Emotional and behavioural effects of participating in an online study of nonsuicidal self-injury: An experimental analysis. *Clinical Psychological Science, 3,* 26–37.

46. Cha, C. B., Glenn, J. J., Deming, C. A., D'Angelo, E. J., Hooley, J. M., Teachman, B. A., & Nock, M. K. (2016). Examining potential iatrogenic effects of viewing suicide and self-injury stimuli. *Psychological Assessment, 28,* 1510–1515.

47. Hasking, P., Tatnell, R., & Martin, G. (2015). Adolescents' reactions to participating in ethically sensitive research: A prospective self-report study. *Child and Adolescent Psychiatry and Mental Health, 9,* 39.

48. Jorm, A. F., Kelly, C. M., & Morgan, A. J. (2007). Participant distress in psychiatric research: A systematic review. *Psychological Medicine, 37,* 917–926.

49. Whitlock, J., Pietrusza, C., & Purrington, A. (2013). Young adult respondent experiences of disclosing self-injury, suicide-related behavior, and psychological distress in a web-based survey. *Archives of Suicide Research, 17,* 20–32.

50. Hasking, P., Lewis, S. P., Robinson, K., Heath, N. L., & Wilson, M. (2019). Conducting research on nonsuicidal self-injury in schools: Ethical considerations and recommendations. *School Psychology International, 40,* 217–234.

51. Lloyd-Richardson E. E., Lewis, S. P., Whitlock, J. L., Rodham, K., & Schatten, H. (2015). Research with adolescents who engage in non-suicidal self-injury: Ethical considerations and challenges. *Child and Adolescent Psychiatry and Mental Health, 9,* 37.

52. Walsh, B. W. (2012). *Treating self-injury: A practical guide* (2nd ed.). Guilford Press.

53. Richardson, B. G., Surmitis, K. A., & Hydahl, R. S. (2012). Minimising social contagion in adolescents who self-injure: Considerations for group work, residential treatment, and the Internet. *Journal of Mental Health Counselling, 34,* 121–132.

Chapter 7

1. Kietzmann, J. H., Hermkens, K., McCarthy, I. P., & Silvestre, B. S. (2011). Social media? Get serious! Understanding the functional building blocks of social media. *Business Horizons, 54,* 241–251. https://doi.org/10.1016/j.bushor.2011.01.005.

2. Pew Research Center. (2018). *Teens, social media and technology 2018.* https://www.pewresearch.org/internet/2018/05/31/teens-social-media-technology-2018/

3. Pew Research Center. (2021). *About three-in-ten U.S. adults say they are "almost constantly" online.* https://www.pewresearch.org/fact-tank/2021/03/26/about-three-in-ten-u-s-adults-say-they-are-almost-constantly-online/).

4. Lewis, S. P., & Seko, Y. (2016). A double-edged sword: A review of benefits and risks of online nonsuicidal self-injury activities. *Journal of Clinical Psychology, 72*(3), 249–262.

5. Dyson, M. P., Hartling, L., Shulhan, J., Chisholm, A., Milne, A., Sundar, P., . . . Newton, A. S. (2016). A systematic review of social media use to discuss and view deliberate self-harm acts. *PLOSOne, 11,* e0155813.

6. Marchant, A., Hawton, K., Stewart, A., Montgomery, P., Singaravelu, V., Lloyd, K., . . . John, A. (2017). A systematic review of the relationship between internet use, self-harm, and suicidal behaviour in young people: The good, the bad, and the unknown. *PLOSOne, 12*, e0181722. https://doi.org/10.1371/journal.pone.0181722.

7. Arendt, F., Scherr, S., & Romer, D. (2019). Effects of exposure to self-harm on social media: Evidence from a two-wave panel study among young adults. *New Media and Society, 21*(11–12), 2422–2442.

8. Lewis, S. P., & Baker, T. G. (2011). The possible risks of self-injury web sites: A content analysis. *Archives of Suicide Research, 15*(4), 390–396.

9. Lewis, S. P., Heath, N. L., St Denis, J. M., & Noble, R. (2011). The scope of nonsuicidal self-injury on YouTube. *Pediatrics, 127*(3), e552–e557.

10. Rowe, S. L., French, R. S., Henderson, C., Ougrin, D., Slade, M., & Morgan, P. (2014). Help-seeking behaviour and adolescent self-harm: A systematic review. *Australian and New Zealand Journal of Psychiatry, 48*, 1083–1095.

11. Whitlock, J. L., Powers, J. L., & Eckenrode, J. (2006). The virtual cutting edge: The internet and adolescent self-injury. *Developmental Psychology, 42*(3), 407.

12. Lewis, S. P., Kenny, T., & Pritchard, T. (2019). Self-injury and the Internet: A review of the evidence and clinical recommendations. In. J. Washburn (Ed.), *Nonsuicidal self-injury: Advances in Research and Practice*. New York.

13. Jacob, N., Evans, R., & Scourfield, J. (2017). The influence of online images on self-harm: A qualitative study of young people aged 16–24. *Journal of Adolescence, 60*, 140–147.

14. Lewis, S. P., & Michal, N. J. (2016). Stop, start, and continue: Preliminary insight into the appeal of self-injury e-communication. *Journal of Health Psychology, 21*, 250–260.

15. Staniland, L., Hasking, P., Boyes, M., & Lewis, S. (2021). Stigma and nonsuicidal self-injury: Application of a conceptual framework. *Stigma and Health, 6*(3), 312.

16. Murray, C. D., & Fox, J. (2006). Do internet self-harm discussion groups alleviate or exacerbate self-harming behaviour? *Australian e-Journal for the Advancement of Mental Health, 5*, 225–233. https://doi.org/10.5172/jamh.5.3.225.

17. Jones, R., Sharkey, S., Ford, T., Emmens, T., Hewis, E., Smithson, J. . . . Owens, C. (2011). Online discussion forums for young people who self-harm: User views. *The Psychiatrist, 35*, 364–368. https://doi.org/10.1192/pb.bp.110.033449.

18. Lewis, S. P., Rosenrot, S. A., & Messner, M. A. (2012). Seeking validation in unlikely places: The nature of online questions about non-suicidal self-injury. *Archives of Suicide Research, 16*, 263–272. https://doi.org/10.1080/13811118.2012.695274.

19. Brown, R. C., Fischer, T., Goldwich, A. D., Keller, F., Young, R., & Plener, P. L. (2018). #Cutting: Non-suicidal self-injury (NSSI) on Instagram. *Psychological Medicine, 48*(2), 337–346.

20. Lewis, S. P., Heath, N. L., Sornberger, M. J., & Arbuthnott, A. E. (2012). Helpful or harmful? An examination of viewers' responses to nonsuicidal self-injury videos on YouTube. *Journal of Adolescent Health, 51*, 380–385.

21. Rodham, K., Gavin, J., Lewis, S. P., St. Denis, J., & Bandalli, P. (2013). An investigation of the motivations driving the online representation of self-injury: A thematic analysis. *Archives of Suicide Research, 17*, 173–183.

22. Sternudd, H. T. (2012). Photographs of self-injury: Production and reception in a group of self-injurers. *Journal of Youth Studies, 15*, 421–436.

23. Haberstroh, S., & Moyer, M. (2012). Exploring an online self-injury support group: Perspectives from group members. *Journal for Specialists in Group Work, 37*, 113–132. https://doi.org/10.1080/01933922.2011.646088.

24. Johnson, G. M., Zastawny, S., & Kulpa, A. (2010). E-message boards for those who self-injure: Implications for E-health. *International Journal of Mental Health and Addiction, 8*, 566–569.

25. Lewis, S. P., Mahdy, J. C., Michal, N. J., & Arbuthnott, A. E. (2014). Googling self-injury: The state of health information obtained through online searches for self-injury. *JAMA Pediatrics, 168*, 443–449.

26. Frost, M., & Casey, L. (2016). Who seeks help online for self-injury? *Archives of Suicide Research, 20*, 69–79.

27. Pritchard, T. R., Lewis, S. P., & Marcincinova, I. (2021). Needs of youth posting about nonsuicidal self-injury: A time-trend analysis. *Journal of Adolescent Health, 68*(3), 532–539.

28. Lewis, S. P., Heath, N. L., Michal, N. J., & Duggan, J. M. (2012). Non-suicidal self-injury, youth, and the internet: What mental health professionals need to know. *Child and Adolescent Psychiatry and Mental Health, 6*(1), 1–9.

29. Mitten, N., Preyde, M., Lewis, S., Vanderkooy, J., & Heintzman, J. (2016). The perceptions of adolescents who self-harm on stigma and care following inpatient psychiatric treatment. *Social Work in Mental Health, 14*(1), 1–21.

30. Rosenrot, S. A., & Lewis, S. P. (2020). Barriers and responses to the disclosure of non-suicidal self-injury: A thematic analysis. *Counselling Psychology Quarterly, 33*(2), 121–141.

31. De Riggi, M. E., Lewis, S. P., & Heath, N. L. (2018). Brief report: Nonsuicidal self-injury in adolescence: Turning to the internet for support. *Counselling Psychology Quarterly, 31*(3), 397–405.

32. Adler, P. A., & Adler, P. (2008). The cyber worlds of self-injurers: Deviant communities, relationships, and selves. *Symbolic Interaction, 31*, 33–56.

33. Baker, D., & Fortune, S. (2008). Understanding self-harm and suicide websites: A qualitative interview study of young adult website users. *Crisis, 29*, 118–122. https://doi.org/10.1027/0227-5910.29.3.118.

34. Niwa, K. D., & Mandrusiak, M. N. (2012). Self-injury groups on Facebook. *Canadian Journal of Counseling and Psychotherapy, 46*, 1–20.

35. Owens, C., Sharkey, S., Smithson, J., Hewis, E., Emmens, T., Ford, T., & Jones, R. (2012). Building an online community to promote communication and collaborative learning between health professionals and young people who self-harm: An exploratory study. *Health Expectations, 18*, 81–94. https://doi.org/10.1111/hex.12011.

36. Rodham, K., Gavin, J., & Miles, M. (2007). I hear, I listen, I care: A qualitative investigation into the function of a self-harm message board. *Suicide and Life-Threatening Behaviour, 37*, 422–430.

37. Saunders, K. E. A., Hawton, K., Fortune, S., & Farrell, S. (2012). Attitudes and knowledge of clinical staff regarding people who self-harm: A systematic review. *Journal of Affective Disorders, 139*, 205–216. https://doi.org/10.1016/j.jad.2011.08.024.

38. Linehan, M. M. (1993). *Cognitive-behavioural treatment of borderline personality disorder*. Guilford Press.

39. Duggan, J. M., Heath, N. L., Lewis, S. P., & Baxter, A. L. (2012). An examination of the scope and nature of non-suicidal self-injury online activities: Implications for

school mental health professionals. *School Mental Health*, *4*, 56–67. https://doi.org/ 10.1007/s12310–011-9065–6.

40. Whitlock, J. L., Powers, J. L., & Eckenrode, J. (2006). The virtual cutting edge: The internet and adolescent self-injury. *Developmental Psychology*, *42*, 407–417. https:// doi.org/10.1037/0012–1649.42.3.407.

41. Lewis, S. P., Seko, Y., & Joshi, P. (2018). The impact of YouTube peer feedback on attitudes toward recovery from non-suicidal self-injury: An experimental pilot study. *Digital Health*, *4*, 2055207618780499.

42. Lewis, S. P., & Knoll, A. K. (2015). Do it yourself: Examination of self-injury first aid tips on YouTube. *Cyberpsychology, Behavior, and Social Networking*, *18*(5), 301–304.

43. Baker, T. G., & Lewis, S. P. (2013). Responses to online photographs of nonsuicidal self-injury: A thematic analysis. *Archives of Suicide Research*, *17*, 223–235. https:// doi.org/10.1080/13811118.2013.805642.

44. Zdanow, C., & Wright, B. (2012). The representation of self injury and suicide on emo social networking groups. *African Sociological Review/ Revue Africaine de Sociologie*, *16*, 81–101.

45. Pritchard, T. R., Fedchenko, C. A., & Lewis, S. P. (2021). Self-injury is my drug: The functions of describing nonsuicidal self-injury as an addiction. *Journal of Nervous and Mental Disease*, *209*(9), 628–635.

46. Cha, C. B., Glenn, J. J., Deming, C. A., D'Angelo, E. J., Hooley, J. M., Teachman, B. A., & Nock, M. K. (2016). Examining potential iatrogenic effects of viewing suicide and self-injury stimuli. *Psychological Assessment*, *28*(11), 1510.

47. Hasking, P., Andrews, T., & Martin, G. (2013). The role of exposure to self-injury among peers in predicting later self-injury. *Journal of Youth and Adolescence*, *42*(10), 1543–1556.

48. Sanson, M., Strange, D., & Garry, M. (2019). Trigger warnings are trivially helpful at reducing negative affect, intrusive thoughts, and avoidance. *Clinical Psychological Science*, *7*(4), 778–793.

49. Swannell, S., Martin, G., Krysinska, K., Kay, T., Olsson, K., & Win, A. (2010). Cutting on-line: Self-injury and the Internet. *Advances in Mental Health*, *9*, 177–189.

50. Lewis, S. P., Bryant, L. A., Schaefer, B. M., & Grunberg, P. H. (2017). In their own words: Perspectives on nonsuicidal self-injury disorder among those with lived experience. *Journal of Nervous and Mental Disease*, *205*(10), 771–779.

51. Walsh, B. W. (2012). *Treating self-injury: A practical guide*. Guilford Press.

52. Kettlewell, C. (1999). *Skin game: A memoir*. Macmillan.

53. Lewis, S. P., & Hasking, P. A. (2021). Understanding self-injury: A person-centered approach. *Psychiatric Services*, *72*(6), 721–723.

54. Westers, N. J., Lewis, S. P., Whitlock, J., Schatten, H. T., Ammerman, B., Andover, M. S., & Lloyd-Richardson, E. E. (2021). Media guidelines for the responsible reporting and depicting of non-suicidal self-injury. *British Journal of Psychiatry*, *219*(2), 415–418.

Chapter 8

1. Martin, G., Richardson, A. S., Bergen, H. A., Roeger, L., & Allison, S. (2005). Perceived academic performance, self-esteem and locus of control as indicators of need for assessment of adolescent suicide risk: Implications for teachers. *Journal of Adolescence*, *28*, 75–87.

2. Monto, M. A., McRee, N., & Deryck, F. S. (2018). Nonsuicidal self-injury among a representative sample of US adolescents. *American Journal of Public Health, 108,* 1042–1048.

3. Madjar, N., Ben Shabat, S., Elia, R., Fellner, N., Rehavi, M., Rubin, S. E., Segal, N., & Shoval, G. (2017a). Non-suicidal self-injury within the school context: Multilevel analysis of teachers' support and peer climate. *European Psychiatry, 41,* 95–101.

4. Madjar, N., Zalsman, G., Ben Mordechai, T. R., & Shoval, G. (2017b). Repetitive vs. occasional non-suicidal self-injury and school-related factors among Israeli high school students. *Psychiatry Research, 257,* 358–360.

5. Perkins, N., de Riggi, M., Hasking, P., & Heath, N. (2022). Slipping through the cracks: The critical role of school principals in addressing and responding to nonsuicidal self-injury among adolescents. *Psychology in the Schools.* https://doi.org/10.1002/pits.22811

6. Hasking, P., Heath, N. L., Kaess, M., Lewis, S. P., Plener, P. L., Walsh, B. W., Whitlock, J., & Wilson, M. S. (2016). Position paper for guiding response to non-suicidal self-injury in schools. *School Psychology International, 37,* 644–663.

7. Lewis, S. P., Heath, N. L., Hasking, P. A., Hamza, C., Bloom, E., Lloyd-Richardson, E., & Whitlock, J. (2020). Advocacy for improved response to self-injury in schools: A call to action for school psychologists. *Psychological Services, 17,* 86–92.

8. Whitlock, J., Lloyd-Richardson, E., Fisseha, F., & Bates, T. (2018). Parental secondary stress: The often hidden consequences of nonsuicidal self-injury in youth. *Journal of Clinical Psychology, 74,* 178–196.

9. Berger, E., Hasking, P., & Reupert, A. (2014). "We're working in the dark here": Knowledge, attitudes and response of school staff towards adolescents' self-injury. *School Mental Health, 6,* 201–212.

10. Roberts-Dobie, S., & Donatelle, R. J. (2007). School counselors and student self-injury. *Journal of School Health, 77,* 257–264.

11. Duggan, J. M., Heath, N. L., Toste, J. R., & Ross, S. (2011). School counsellors' understanding of nonsuicidal self-injury: Experiences and international variability. *Canadian Journal of Counselling and Psychotherapy, 45,* 327–348.

12. Kelada, L., Hasking, P., & Melvin, G. (2017). School response to self-injury: Concerns of mental health staff and parents. *School Psychology Quarterly, 32,* 173–187.

13. Kelada, L., Hasking, P., & Melvin, G. (2016). The relationship between nonsuicidal self-injury and family functioning: Adolescent and parent perspectives. *Journal of Marital and Family Therapy, 42,* 536–549.

14. Berger, E., Hasking, P., & Martin, G. (2017). Adolescents' perspectives of youth non-suicidal self-injury prevention. *Youth and Society, 49,* 3–22.

15. Berger, E., Hasking, P., & Reupert, P. (2014). Response and training needs of school staff towards students' self-injury. *Teaching and Teacher Education, 44,* 25–34.

16. Heath, N. L., Toste, J. R., & Beettam, E. L. (2006). "I am not well-equipped": High school teachers' perceptions of self-injury. *Canadian Journal of School Psychology, 21,* 73–92.

17. Heath, N. L., Toste, J. R., Sornberger, M. J., & Wagner, C. (2011). Teachers' perceptions of non-suicidal self-injury in the schools. *School Mental Health, 3,* 35–43.

18. Gandhi, A., Luyckx, K., Goossens, L., Maitra, S., & Claes, L. (2018). Association between non-suicidal self-injury, parents and peer related loneliness and attitudes toward aloneness in Flemish adolescents: An empirical note. *Psychologica Belgica, 58,* 3–12.

19. Tatnell, R., Kelada, L., Hasking, P., & Martin, G. (2014). Longitudinal analysis of adolescent NSSI: The role of intrapersonal and interpersonal factors. *Journal of Abnormal Child Psychology, 42*, 885–896.

20. White Kress, V. E., Costin, A., & Drouhard, N. (2006). Students who self-injure: School counsellor ethical and legal considerations. *Professional School Counselling, 10*, 203–209.

21. Arbuthnott, A. E., & Lewis, S. P. (2015). Parents of youth who self-injure: A review of the literature and implications for mental health professionals. *Child and Adolescent Psychiatry and Mental Health, 9*(1), 1–20.

22. Whitlock, J., Lloyd-Richardson, E., Fisseha, F., & Bates, T. (2018). Parental secondary stress: The often hidden consequences of non-suicidal self-injury in youth. *Journal of Clinical Psychology, 74*, 178–196.

23. Whitlock, J., Baetens, I., Lloyd-Richardson, E., Hasking, P., Hamza, C., Lewis, S. P., Franz, P., & Robinson, K. (2018). Helping schools support parents of youth who self-injure: Considerations and recommendations. *School Psychology International, 39*, 312–328.

24. Kelada, L., Whitlock, J., Hasking, P., & Melvin, G. (2016). Parents' experiences of nonsuicidal self-injury among adolescents and young adults. *Journal of Child and Family Studies, 25*, 3403–3416.

25. Victor, S., Hipwell, A. E., Stepp, S. D., & Scott, L. N. (2019). Parent and peer relationships as longitudinal predictors of adolescent non-suicidal self-injury onset. *Child and Adolescent Psychiatry and Mental Health, 13*(1), 1–13.

26. Xavier, A., Pinto Gouveia, J., & Cunha, M. (2016, August). Non-suicidal self-injury in adolescence: The role of shame, self-criticism and fear of self-compassion. In *Child & youth care forum* (Vol. 45, No. 4, pp. 571–586). Springer.

27. Fisher, K., Fitzgerald, J., & Tuffin, K. (2017). Peer responses to non-suicidal self-injury: Young women speak about the complexity of the support-provider role. *New Zealand Journal of Psychology, 46*, 146–155.

28. Jorm, A. F., Kelly, C. M., & Morgan, A. J. (2007). Participant distress in psychiatric research: A systematic review. *Psychological Medicine, 37*(7), 917–926.

29. Robinson, J., Gook, S., Yuen, H. P., McGorry, P. D., & Yung, A. R. (2008). Managing deliberate self-harm in young people: An evaluation of a training program developed for school welfare staff using a longitudinal research design. *BMC Psychiatry, 8*, 75.

30. Wyman, P. A., Brown, C. H., Inman, J., Cross, W., Schmeelk-Cone, K., Guo, J., Pena, J. B. (2008). Randomized trial of a gatekeeper program for suicide prevention: 1-year impact on secondary school staff. *Journal of Consulting and Clinical Psychology, 76*, 104–115.

31. Groschwitz, R., Munz, L., Straub, J., Bohnacker, I., & Plener, P. L. (2017). Strong schools against suicidality and self-injury: Evaluation of a workshop for school staff. *School Psychology Quarterly, 32*, 188–198.

32. McAllister, M., Hasking, P. A., Estefan, A., McClenaghan, K., & Lowe, J. (2010). A strengths-based group program on self-harm: A feasibility study. *Journal of School Nursing, 26*, 289–300.

33. Hasking, P., Baetens, I., Bloom, E., Heath, N., Lewis, S., Lloyd-Richardson, E., & Robinson, K. (2019). Addressing and responding to nonsuicidal self-injury in the school context. In J. Washburn (Ed.), *Nonsuicidal self-injury: Advances in research and practice* (pp. 175–194). Routledge.

34. Baker, T. G., & Lewis, S. P. (2013). Responses to online photographs of non-suicidal self-injury: A thematic analysis. *Archives of Suicide Research, 17*, 223–235.

35. Lewis, S. P. (2016). The overlooked role of self-injury scars: A commentary and suggestions for clinical practice. *Journal of Nervous and Mental Disease, 204*, 33–35.

36. Lewis, S. P., & Mehrabkhani, S. (2016). Every scar tells a story: Insight into people's self-injury scar experiences. *Counselling Psychology Quarterly, 29*, 296–310.

37. Hasking, P., & Boyes, M. (2018). Cutting words: A commentary on language and stigma in the context of non-suicidal self-injury. *Journal of Nervous and Mental Disease, 206*, 829–833.

38. Lewis, S. P., & Seko, Y. (2016). A double-edged sword: A review of benefits and risks of online nonsuicidal self-injury activities. *Journal of Clinical Psychology, 72*, 249–262.

39. Radovic, S., & Hasking, P. (2013). The relationship between film portrayals of non-suicidal self-injury, attitudes, knowledge and behaviour. *Crisis, 34*, 324–334.

40. Trewavas, C., Hasking, P. A., & McAllister, M. (2010). Representations of non-suicidal self-injury in motion pictures. *Archives of Suicide Research, 14*, 89–103.

41. Cha, C. B., Glenn, J. J., Deming, C. A., D'Angelo, E. J., Hooley, J. M., Teachman, B. A., & Nock, M. K. (2016). Examining potential iatrogenic effects of viewing suicide and self-injury stimuli. *Psychological Assessment, 28*, 1510–1515.

42. Hasking, P., Andrews, T., & Martin, G. (2013). The role of exposure to self-injury among peers in predicting later self-injury. *Journal of Youth and Adolescence, 42*, 1543–1556.

43. Hasking, P., & Rose, A. (2016). A preliminary application of social cognitive theory to nonsuicidal self-injury. *Journal of Youth and Adolescence, 45*, 1560–1574.

44. De Riggi, M. E., Moumne, S., Heath, N. L., & Lewis, S. P. (2017). Non-suicidal self-injury in our schools: A review and research-informed guidelines for school mental health professionals. *Canadian Journal of School Psychology, 32*, 122–143.

Chapter 9

1. Victor, S. E., Hipwell, A. E., Stepp, S. D., & Scott, L. N. (2019). Parent and peer relationships as longitudinal predictors of adolescent non-suicidal self-injury onset. *Child and Adolescent Psychiatry and Mental Health, 13*, 1.

2. Tatnell, R., Kelada, L., Hasking, P., & Martin, G. (2014). Longitudinal analysis of adolescent NSSI: The role of intrapersonal and interpersonal factors. *Journal of Abnormal Child Psychology, 42*, 885–896.

3. Turner, B. J., Wakefield, M. A., Gratz, K. L., & Chapman, A. L. (2017). Characterizing interpersonal difficulties among young adults who engage in non-suicidal self-injury using a daily diary. *Behaviour Therapy, 48*, 366–379.

4. Taliaferrio, L. A., McMorris, B. J., Rider, G. N., & Eisenberg, M. E. (2019). Risk and protective factors for self-harm in a population-based sample of transgender youth. *Archives of Suicide Research, 23*, 203–221.

5. Taliaferro, L. A., Jang, S. T., Westers, N. J., Meuhlenkamp, J. J., Whitlock, J. L., & McMorris, B. J. (2020). Associations between connections to parents and friends and non-suicidal self-injury among adolescents: The mediating role of developmental assets. *Clinical Child Psychology and Psychiatry, 25*, 359–371.

6. Brausch, A. M., & Gutierrez, P. M. (2010). Differences in non-suicidal self-injury and suicide attempts in adolescents. *Journal of Youth and Adolescence, 39*, 233–242.

7. Hasking, P., Rees, C., Martin, G., & Quigley, J. (2015). What happens when you tell someone you self-injure? The effects of disclosing NSSI to adults and peers. *BMC Public Health, 15*, 1039.

8. James, K. M., & Gibb, B. E. (2019). Maternal criticism and non-suicidal self-injury in school-aged children. *Psychiatry Research, 273*, 89–93.

9. Cassels, M., van Harmelen, A., Neufeld, S., Goodyer, I., Jones, P. B., & Wilkinson, P. (2018). Poor family functioning mediates the link between childhood adversity and adolescent nonsuicidal self-injury. *Journal of Child Psychology and Psychiatry, 59*, 881–887.

10. Wolff, J., Frazier, E. A., Esposito-Smythers, C., Burke, T., Sloan, E., & Spirito, A. (2013). Cognitive and social factors associated with NSSI and suicide attempts in psychiatrically hospitalised adolescents. *Journal of Abnormal Child Psychology, 41*, 1005–1013.

11. Hasking, P., Dawkins, J., Gray, N., Wijeratne, P., & Boyes, M. (2020). Indirect effects of family functioning on NSSI and risky drinking: The roles of emotion reactivity and emotion regulation. *Journal of Child and Family Studies, 29*, 2070–2079.

12. Dawkins, J., Hasking, P., & Boyes, M. (2019). Knowledge of parental nonsuicidal self-injury in young people who self-injure: The mediating role of outcome expectancies. *Journal of Family Studies, 27*(4), 479–490.

13. Baetens, I., Claes, L., Martin, G., Onghena, P., Grietens, H. Van Leeuwen, K., Pieters, C., Wiersema, J. R., & Griffith, J. W. (2014). Is nonsuicidal self-injury associated with parenting and family factors? *Journal of Early Adolescence, 34*, 387–405.

14. Kelada, L., Hasking, P., & Melvin, G. (2016). The relationship between nonsuicidal self-injury and family functioning: Adolescent and parent perspectives. *Journal of Marital and Family Therapy, 42*, 536–549.

15. Arbuthnott, A. E., & Lewis, S. P. (2015). Parents of youth who self-injure: A review of the literature and implications for mental health professionals. *Child and Adolescent Psychiatry and Mental Health, 9*, 35.

16. Liu, R. T., Scopelliti, K. M., Pittman, S. K., & Zamora, A. S. (2018). Childhood maltreatment and non-suicidal self-injury: A systematic review and meta-analysis. *Lancet Psychiatry, 5*, 51–64.

17. Lang, C. M., & Sharma-Patel, K. (2011). The relation between childhood maltreatment and self-injury: A review of the literature on conceptualisation and intervention. *Trauma, Violence, and Abuse, 12*, 23–37.

18. Swannell, S., Martin, G., Page, A., Hasking, P., Hazell, P., Taylor, A., & Protani, M. (2012). Child maltreatment, subsequent non-suicidal self-injury and the mediating roles of dissociation, alexithymia and self-blame. *Child Abuse and Neglect, 36*, 572–584.

19. Linehan, M. (1993). *Cognitive-behavioral treatment of borderline personality disorder*. Guilford Press.

20. Crowell, S. E., Beauchaine, T. P., & Linehan, M. M. (2009). A biosocial developmental model of borderline personality: Elaborating and extending Linehan's theory. *Psychological Bulletin, 135*, 495–510.

21. Shore, A. N. (2000). Attachment and the regulation of the right brain. *Attachment and Human Development, 2*, 23–47.

22. Gandhi, A., Luyckx, K., Molenberghs, G., Baetens, I., Goossens, L., Maitra, S., & Claes, L. (2019). Maternal and peer attachment, identity formation, and non-suicidal self-injury: A longitudinal mediation study. *Child and Adolescent Psychiatry and Mental Health, 13*, 7.

23. Fonagy, P., Steele, M., Steele, H., Moran, G. S., & Higgitt, A. C. (1991). The capacity for understanding mental states: The reflective self in parent and child and its significance for security of attachment. *Infant Mental Health Journal, 12*, 201–218.

24. Fonagy, P., & Target, M. (1997). Attachment and reflective function: Their role in self-organisation. *Development and Psychopathology, 9*, 679–700.

25. Cucchi, A., Hampton, J. A., & Moulton-Perkins, A. (2018). Using the validated Reflective Functioning Questionnaire to investigate mentalizing in individuals presenting with eating disorders and with and without self-harm. *PeerJ, 6*:e5756.

26. Badoud, D., Luyten, P., Fonseca-Pedrero, E., Eliez, S., Fonagy, P., & Debbane, M. (2015). The French version of the Reflective Functioning Questionnaire: Validity data for adolescents and adults and its association with non-suicidal self-injury. *PLOSOne, 10*, e0145892.

27. Kim, S., Fonagy, P., Allen, J., & Strathearn, L. (2014). Mothers' unresolved trauma blunts amygdala response to infant distress. *Social Neuroscience, 9*, 352–363.

28. Kissil, K. (2011). Attachment-based family therapy for adolescent self-injury. *Journal of Family Psychotherapy, 22*, 313–327.

29. Cook, N. E., & Gorraiz, M. (2016). Dialectical behavior therapy for nonsuicidal self-injury and depression among adolescents: Preliminary meta-analytic evidence. *Child and Adolescent Mental Health, 2*, 81–89.

30. Hoffman, P. D., Fruzetti, A. E., & Swenson, C. R. (1999). Dialectical behaviour therapy—family skills training. *Family Processes, 38*, 399–414.

31. Bateman, A., & Fonagy, P. (2013). Mentalization-based treatment. *Journal of Mental Health Professionals, 33*, 595–613.

32. Rossouw, T. I., & Fonagy, P. (2012). Metallization-based treatment for self-harm in adolescents: A randomised controlled trial. *Journal of the American Academy of Child and Adolescent Psychiatry, 51*, 1304–1313.

33. Barnicot, K., & Crawford, M. (2019). Dialectical behaviour therapy v. mentalisation-based therapy for borderline personality disorder. *Psychological Medicine, 49*, 2060–2068.

34. Slade, A. (2007). Reflective parenting programs: Theory and development. *Psychoanalytic Inquiry, 26*, 640–657.

35. Asen, E., & Fonagy, P. (2012). Mentalization-based therapeutic interventions for families. *Journal of Family Therapy, 34*, 347–370.

36. Hoffman, R., Hinkel. M. G., & Kress, V. W. (2010). Letter writing intervention in family therapy with adolescents who engage in nonsuicidal self-injury. *Family Journal: Counselling and Therapy for Couples and Families, 18*, 24–30.

37. Schade, L. C. (2013). Non-suicidal self-injury (NSSI): A case for using emotionally focused family therapy. *Contemporary Family Therapy, 35*, 568–582.

38. Kelada, L., Whitlock, J., Hasking, P., & Melvin, G. (2016). Parents' experiences of nonsuicidal self-injury among adolescents and young adults. *Journal of Child and Family Studies, 25*, 3403–3416.

39. Whitlock, J., Lloyd-Richardson, E., Fisseha, F., & Bates, T. (2018). Parental secondary stress: The often hidden consequences of non-suicidal self-injury in youth. *Journal of Clinical Psychology, 74*, 178–196.

40. Whitlock, J., & Lloyd-Richardson, E. (2019). *Healing self-injury: A compassionate guide for parents and other loved ones.* Oxford University Press.

41. Baetens, I., Claes, L., Onghena, P., Grietens, H., van Leeuwen, K., Pieters, C., Wiersema, J. R., & Griffith, J. W. (2015). The effects of nonsuicidal self-injury on parenting behaviours: A longitudinal analysis of the perspective of the parent. *Child and Adolescent Psychiatry and Mental Health, 9,* 24.

42. Waals, L., Baetens, I., Rober, P., Lewis, S., van Parys, H., Goethals, E. R., & Whitlock, J. (2018). The NSSI family distress cascade theory. *Child and Adolescent Psychiatry and Mental Health, 12,* 52.

43. Berger, E., Hasking, P., & Martin, G. (2013). "Listen to them": Adolescents' views on helping young people who self-injure. *Journal of Adolescence, 36,* 935–945.

44. Walsh, B., & Walsh, B. W. (2005). *Treating self-injury: A practical guide.* Guilford Press.

45. Tschan, T., Lüdtke, J., Schmid, M., & In-Albon, T. (2019). Sibling relationships of female adolescents with nonsuicidal self-injury disorder in comparison to a clinical and a nonclinical control group. *Child and Adolescent Psychiatry and Mental Health, 13,* 15.

Chapter 10

1. Klonsky, E. D., & Lewis, S. P. (2014). Assessment of non-suicidal self-injury. In M. K. Nock (Ed.), *Oxford handbook of suicide and self-injury* (pp. 337–354). Oxford University Press.

2. Walsh, B. (2007). Clinical assessment of self-injury: A practical guide. *Journal of Clinical Psychology, 63*(11), 1057–1068.

3. Walsh, B. W. (2012). *Treating self-injury: A practical guide.* Guilford Press.

4. Kettlewell, C. (1999). *Skin game: A cutter's memoir.* St. Martin's Press.

5. Klonsky, E. D., Muehlenkamp, J., Lewis, S. P., & Walsh, B. (2011). *Nonsuicidal self-injury* (Vol. 22). Hogrefe Publishing.

6. Washburn, J. J., Richardt, S. L., Styer, D. M., Gebhardt, M., Juzwin, K. R., Yourek, A., & Aldridge, D. (2012). Psychotherapeutic approaches to non-suicidal self-injury in adolescents. *Child and Adolescent Psychiatry and Mental Health, 6*(1), 1–8.

7. Andover, M. S., Holman, C. S., & Shashoua, M. Y. (2014). Functional assessment of non-suicidal self-injury and eating disorders. In Laurence Claes & Jennifer J. Muehlenkamp (Eds.), *Non-suicidal self-injury in eating disorders* (pp. 87–104). Springer.

8. Rizvi, S. L. (2019). *Chain analysis in dialectical behavior therapy.* Guilford Publications.

9. Linehan, M. M. (1993). *Cognitive-behavioral treatment of borderline personality disorder.* Guilford Publications.

10. Glenn, C. R., Franklin, J. C., & Nock, M. K. (2015). Evidence-based psychosocial treatments for self-injurious thoughts and behaviors in youth. *Journal of Clinical Child and Adolescent Psychology, 44*(1), 1–29.

11. Turner, B. J., Austin, S. B., & Chapman, A. L. (2014). Treating nonsuicidal self-injury: A systematic review of psychological and pharmacological interventions. *Canadian Journal of Psychiatry, 59*(11), 576–585.

12. Miller, A. L., Rathus, J. H., DuBose, A. P., Dexter-Mazza, E. T., & Goldklang, A. R. (2007). Dialectical behavior therapy for adolescents. *Dialectical Behavior Therapy in Clinical Practice: Applications Across Disorders and Settings,* 245–263.

13. Rathus, J. H., & Miller, A. L. (2014). *DBT skills manual for adolescents*. Guilford Publications.

14. Lewis, S. P., & Heath, N. L. (2015). Nonsuicidal self-injury among youth. *Journal of Pediatrics, 166*(3), 526–530.

15. Swannell, S. V., Martin, G. E., Page, A., Hasking, P., & St John, N. J. (2014). Prevalence of nonsuicidal self-injury in nonclinical samples: Systematic review, meta-analysis and meta-regression. *Suicide and Life-Threatening Behavior, 44*(3), 273–303.

16. Waals, L., Baetens, I., Rober, P., Lewis, S., Van Parys, H., Goethals, E. R., & Whitlock, J. (2018). The NSSI family distress cascade theory. *Child and Adolescent Psychiatry and Mental Health, 12*(1), 1–6.

17. Baetens, I., Claes, L., Martin, G., Onghena, P., Grietens, H., Van Leeuwen, K., . . . Griffith, J. W. (2014). Is nonsuicidal self-injury associated with parenting and family factors? *Journal of Early Adolescence, 34*(3), 387–405.

18. Baetens, I., Andrews, T., Claes, L., & Martin, G. (2015). The association between family functioning and NSSI in adolescence: The mediating role of depressive symptoms. *Family Science, 6*(1), 330–337.

19. Kress, V. E., & Hoffman, R. M. (2008). Non-suicidal self-injury and motivational interviewing: Enhancing readiness for change. *Journal of Mental Health Counseling, 30*(4), 311–329.

20. Grunberg, P. H., & Lewis, S. P. (2015). Self-injury and readiness to recover: Preliminary examination of components of the stages of change model. *Counselling Psychology Quarterly, 28*(4), 361–371.

21. Kress, V. E., & Hoffman, R. M. (2008). Non-suicidal self-injury and motivational interviewing: Enhancing readiness for change. *Journal of Mental Health Counseling, 30*(4), 311–329.

22. Miller, W. R., & Rollnick, S. (2012). *Motivational interviewing: Helping people change*. Guilford Press.

23. Gratz, K. L., & Gunderson, J. G. (2006). Preliminary data on an acceptance-based emotion regulation group intervention for deliberate self-harm among women with borderline personality disorder. *Behavior Therapy, 37*(1), 25–35.

24. Gratz, K. L., & Tull, M. T. (2011). Extending research on the utility of an adjunctive emotion regulation group therapy for deliberate self-harm among women with borderline personality pathology. *Personality Disorders: Theory, Research, and Treatment, 2*(4), 316.

25. Sahlin, H., Bjureberg, J., Gratz, K. L., Tull, M. T., Hedman, E., Bjärehed, J., . . . Hellner, C. (2017). Emotion regulation group therapy for deliberate self-harm: A multi-site evaluation in routine care using an uncontrolled open trial design. *BMJ Open, 7*(10), e016220.

26. Van Vliet, K., & Kalnins, G. (2011). A compassion-focused approach to nonsuicidal self-injury. *Journal of Mental Health Counseling, 33*(4), 295–311.

27. Sutherland, O., Dawczyk, A., De Leon, K., Cripps, J., & Lewis, S. P. (2014). Self-compassion in online accounts of nonsuicidal self-injury: An interpretive phenomenological analysis. *Counselling Psychology Quarterly, 27*(4), 409–433.

28. Lewis, S. P., Kenny, T. E., Whitfield, K., & Gomez, J. (2019). Understanding self-injury recovery: Views from individuals with lived experience. *Journal of Clinical Psychology, 75*(12), 2119–2139.

29. Kaess, M., Hooley, J. M., Klimes-Dougan, B., Koenig, J., Plener, P. L., Reichl, C., . . . Cullen, K. R. (2021). Advancing a temporal framework for understanding the biology of nonsuicidal self-injury: An expert review. *Neuroscience and Biobehavioral Reviews, 130*, 228–239.

30. Groschwitz, R. C., & Plener, P. L. (2012). The neurobiology of non-suicidal self-injury (NSSI): A review. *Suicidology Online, 3*(1), 24–32.

31. Nixon, M. K., & Heath, N. L. (Eds.). (2008). *Self-injury in youth: The essential guide to assessment and intervention.* Taylor & Francis.

32. Garisch, J. A., Wilson, M. S., O'Connell, A., & Robinson, K. (2017). Overview of assessment and treatment of nonsuicidal self-injury among adolescents. *New Zealand Journal of Psychology (Online), 46*(3), 98–105.

33. Kendall, T., Taylor, C., Bhatti, H., Chan, M., & Kapur, N. (2011). Longer term management of self harm: Summary of NICE guidance. *BMJ, 343,* 7073.

34. Hasking, P. A., Heath, N. L., Kaess, M., Lewis, S. P., Plener, P. L., Walsh, B. W., . . . Wilson, M. S. (2016). Position paper for guiding response to non-suicidal self-injury in schools. *School Psychology International, 37*(6), 644–663.

35. Lewis, S. P., Heath, N. L., Hasking, P. A., Whitlock, J. L., Wilson, M. S., & Plener, P. L. (2019). Addressing self-injury on college campuses: Institutional recommendations. *Journal of College Counseling, 22*(1), 70–82.

36. Wadman, R., Nielsen, E., O'Raw, L., Brown, K., Williams, A. J., Sayal, K., & Townsend, E. (2020). "These things don't work." Young people's views on harm minimization strategies as a proxy for self-harm: A mixed methods approach. *Archives of Suicide Research, 24*(3), 384–401.

Chapter 11

1. Lewis, S. P., & Seko, Y. (2016). A double-edged sword: A review of benefits and risks of online nonsuicidal self-injury activities. *Journal of Clinical Psychology, 72*(3), 249–262.

2. Lewis, S. P. (2016b). Cutting through the shame. *CMAJ: Canadian Medical Association Journal, 188*(17–18), 1265.

3. Ryan-Vig, S., Gavin, J., & Rodham, K. (2019). The presentation of self-harm recovery: A thematic analysis of YouTube videos. *Deviant Behaviour, 40,* 1596–1608.

4. Hasking, P. A., Boyes, M. E., & Lewis, S. P. (2021). The language of self-injury: A data-informed commentary. *Journal of Nervous and Mental Disease, 209*(4), 233–236.

5. Hasking, P., & Boyes, M. (2018). Cutting words: A commentary on language and stigma in the context of nonsuicidal self-injury. *Journal of Nervous and Mental Disease, 206*(11), 829–833.

6. Lewis, S. P. (2017). I cut therefore I am? Avoiding labels in the context of self-injury. *Medical Humanities, 43*(3), 204.

7. Buser, T. J., Pitchko, A., & Buser, J. K. (2014). Naturalistic recovery from nonsuicidal self-injury: A phenomenological inquiry. *Journal of Counseling and Development, 92*(4), 438–446.

8. Lewis, S. P., Seko, Y., & Joshi, P. (2018). The impact of YouTube peer feedback on attitudes toward recovery from non-suicidal self-injury: An experimental pilot study. *Digital Health, 4,* 2055207618780499.

9. Lewis, S. P., Kenny, T. E., Whitfield, K., & Gomez, J. (2019). Understanding self-injury recovery: Views from individuals with lived experience. *Journal of Clinical Psychology, 75*(12), 2119–2139.

10. Whitlock, J., & Lloyd-Richardson, E. E. (2019). *Healing self-injury: A compassionate guide for parents and other loved ones.* Oxford University Press.

11. Lewis, S. P., & Hasking, P. A. (2020). Rethinking self-injury recovery: A commentary and conceptual reframing. *BJPsych Bulletin, 44*(2), 44–46.

12. Lewis, S. P., & Hasking, P. A. (2021). Self-injury recovery: A person-centered framework. *Journal of Clinical Psychology, 77*(4), 884–895.

13. Muehlenkamp, J. J. (2005). Self-injurious behavior as a separate clinical syndrome. *American Journal of Orthopsychiatry, 75*(2), 324–333.

14. American Psychiatric Association. (2013). *Diagnostic and Statistical Manual* (5th ed.). American Psychiatric Association.

15. Hooley, J. M., Fox, K. R., & Boccagno, C. (2020). Nonsuicidal self-injury: Diagnostic challenges and current perspectives. *Neuropsychiatric Disease and Treatment, 16*, 101.

16. Lewis, S. P., Bryant, L. A., Schaefer, B. M., & Grunberg, P. H. (2017). In their own words: Perspectives on nonsuicidal self-injury disorder among those with lived experience. *Journal of Nervous and Mental Disease, 205*(10), 771–779.

17. Prochaska, J. O., & DiClemente, C. C. (1983). Stages and processes of self-change of smoking: Toward an integrative model of change. *Journal of Consulting and Clinical Psychology, 51*(3), 390.

18. Grunberg, P. H., & Lewis, S. P. (2015). Self-injury and readiness to recover: Preliminary examination of components of the stages of change model. *Counselling Psychology Quarterly, 28*(4), 361–371.

19. Kruzan, K. P., Whitlock, J., & Hasking, P. (in press). Development and initial validation of scales to assess decision balance (NSSI-DB), processes of change (NSSI-POC) and self-efficacy (NSSI-SE) in a population of young adults engaging in non-suicidal self-injury. *Psychological Assessment.*

20. Kruzan, K. P., Whitlock, J., & Hasking, P. (2020). Development and initial validation of scales to assess Decisional Balance (NSSI-DB), Processes of Change (NSSI-POC), and Self-Efficacy (NSSI-SE) in a population of young adults engaging in nonsuicidal self-injury. *Psychological Assessment, 32*(7), 635–648.

21. Kelada, L., Hasking, P., Melvin, G., Whitlock, J., & Baetens, I. (2018). "I do want to stop, at least I think I do": An international comparison of recovery from nonsuicidal self-injury among young people. *Journal of Adolescent Research, 33*, 416–441.

22. Gray, N., Hasking, P., & Boyes, M. E. (2021). The impact of ambivalence on recovery from non-suicidal self-injury: Considerations for health professionals. *Journal of Public Mental Health, 20*(4), 251–258.

23. DiClemente, C. C., & Velasquez, M. M. (2002). Motivational interviewing and the stages of change. *Motivational Interviewing: Preparing People for Change, 2*, 201–216.

24. Kruzan, K. P., & Whitlock, J. (2019). Processes of change and nonsuicidal self-injury: A qualitative interview study with individuals at various stages of change. *Global Qualitative Nursing Research, 6*, 1–15.

25. Lewis, S. P., & Mehrabkhani, S. (2016). Every scar tells a story: Insight into people's self-injury scar experiences. *Counselling Psychology Quarterly, 29*(3), 296–310.

26. Long, M. (2018). "We're not monsters . . . we're just really sad sometimes": Hidden self-injury, stigma and help-seeking. *Health Sociology Review, 27*(1), 89–103.

27. Hasking, P., Boyes, M., & Greves, S. (2018). Self-efficacy and emotionally dysregulated behaviour: An exploratory test of the role of emotion regulatory and behaviour-specific beliefs. *Psychiatry Research, 270*, 335–340.

28. Dawkins, J. C., Hasking, P. A., & Boyes, M. E. (2022). Development and validation of a measure of self-efficacy to resist nonsuicidal self-injury. *Journal of Psychopathology and Behavioral Assessment, 44*(2), 511–526.

29. Dawkins, J. C., Hasking, P. A., & Boyes, M. E. (2021). Thoughts and beliefs about nonsuicidal self-injury: An application of social cognitive theory. *Journal of American college health, 69*(4), 428–434.

30. Dawkins, J., Hasking, P., Boyes, M., Greene, D., & Passchier, C. (2019). Applying a cognitive-emotional model to nonsuicidal self-injury. *Stress and Health, 35*, 39–48.

31. Kiekens, G., Hasking, P., Nock, M. K., Boyes, M. E., Kirtley, O., Bruffaerts, R., Myin-Germeys, I., & Claes, L. (2020). Fluctuations in affective states and self-efficacy to resist non-suicidal self-injury as real-time predictors of non-suicidal self-injurious thoughts and behaviours. *Frontiers in Psychiatry, 11*, 214.

32. Heath, N. L., Joly, M., & Carsley, D. (2016). Coping self-efficacy and mindfulness in non-suicidal self-injury. *Mindfulness, 7*(5), 1132–1141.

33. Favazza, A. R., & Rosenthal, R. J. (1993). Diagnostic issues in self-mutilation. *Psychiatric Services, 44*(2), 134–140.

34. Linehan, M. M. (2018). *Cognitive-behavioral treatment of borderline personality disorder*. Guilford Publications.

35. Guérin-Marion, C., Martin, J., Lafontaine, M. F., & Bureau, J. F. (2020). Invalidating caregiving environments, specific emotion regulation deficits, and non-suicidal self-injury. *Child Psychiatry and Human Development, 51*(1), 39–47.

36. Gratz, K. L., & Gunderson, J. G. (2006). Preliminary data on an acceptance-based emotion regulation group intervention for deliberate self-harm among women with borderline personality disorder. *Behavior Therapy, 37*(1), 25–35.

37. Burke, T. A., Olino, T. M., & Alloy, L. B. (2017). Initial psychometric validation of the non-suicidal self-injury scar cognition scale. *Journal of Psychopathology and Behavioral Assessment, 39*(3), 546–562.

38. Lewis, S. P. (2016). The overlooked role of self-injury scars: Commentary and suggestions for clinical practice. *Journal of Nervous and Mental Disease, 204*(1), 33–35.

39. Staniland, L., Hasking, P., Boyes, M., & Lewis, S. (2021). Stigma and nonsuicidal self-injury: Application of a conceptual framework. *Stigma and Health, 6*(3), 312.

40. Rosenrot, S. A., & Lewis, S. P. (2020). Barriers and responses to the disclosure of non-suicidal self-injury: A thematic analysis. *Counselling Psychology Quarterly, 33*(2), 121–141.

41. Hasking, P., Rees, C. S., Martin, G., & Quigley, J. (2015). What happens when you tell someone you self-injure? The effects of disclosing NSSI to adults and peers. *BMC Public Health, 15*(1), 1–9.

42. Sutherland, O., Dawczyk, A., De Leon, K., Cripps, J., & Lewis, S. P. (2014). Self-compassion in online accounts of nonsuicidal self-injury: An interpretive phenomenological analysis. *Counselling Psychology Quarterly, 27*(4), 409–433.

Chapter 12

1. Schwarzer, R. (2008). Modeling health behavior change: How to predict and modify the adoption and maintenance of health behaviors. *Applied Psychology, 57*, 1–29.
2. Marlatt, G. A., & Gordon, J. R. (1985). *Relapse prevention*. Guilford.
3. Hooley, J. M., & Franklin, J. C. (2018). Why do people hurt themselves? A new conceptual model of nonsuicidal self-injury. *Clinical Psychological Science, 6*, 428–451.
4. Gray, N., Hasking, P., & Boyes, M. E. (2021). The impact of ambivalence on recovery from non-suicidal self-injury: Considerations for health professionals. *Journal of Public Mental Health, 20*(4), 251–258.
5. Miller, W. R., & Rollnick, S. (1991). *Motivational interviewing: Preparing people to change addictive behavior*. Guilford Press.
6. Miller, W. R., & Rollnick, S. (2009). Ten things motivational interviewing is not. *Behavioural and Cognitive Psychotherapy, 37*, 129–140.
7. Miller, W. R., & Rose, G. S. (2015). Motivational interviewing and decisional balance: Contrasting responses to client ambivalence. *Behavioural and Cognitive Psychotherapy, 43*, 129–141.
8. Bandura, A. (1977). Self-efficacy: Towards a unifying theory of behavioural change. *Psychological Review, 84*, 191–215.
9. Bandura, A. (1997). *Self-efficacy: The exercise of self-control*. Freeman.
10. Hasking, P., Whitlock, J., Voon, D., & Rose, A. (2017). A cognitive-emotional model of NSSI: Using emotion regulation and cognitive processes to explain why people self-injure. *Cognition and Emotion, 31*, 1543–1556.
11. Dawkins, J., Hasking, P., Boyes, M., Greene, D., & Passchier, C. (2019). Applying a cognitive-emotional model to nonsuicidal self-injury. *Stress and Health, 35*, 39–48.
12. Dawkins, J., Hasking, P., & Boyes, M. (2021). Thoughts and beliefs about nonsuicidal self-injury: An application of social cognitive theory. *Journal of American College Health, 69*, 428–434.
13. Buser, T. J., Buser, J. K., & Kearney, A. (2012). Justice in the family: The moderating role of social self-efficacy in the relationship between nonsuicidal self-injury and interactional justice from parents. *Family Journal, 20*, 147–156.
14. Heath, N. L., Joly, M., & Carsley, D. (2016). Coping self-efficacy and mindfulness in non-suicidal self-injury. *Mindfulness, 7*, 1132–1141.
15. Tatnell, R., Kelada, L., Hasking, P., & Martin, G. (2014). Longitudinal analysis of adolescent NSSI: The role of intrapersonal and interpersonal factors. *Journal of Abnormal Child Psychology, 42*, 885–896.
16. Kelada, L., Hasking, P., Melvin, G., Whitlock, J., & Baetens, I. (2018). "I want to stop, at least I think I do": An international comparison of recovery from nonsuicidal self-injury among young people. *Journal of Adolescent Research, 33*, 416–441.
17. Lewis, S. P., Kenny, T. E., Whitfield, K., & Gomez, J. (2019). Understanding self-injury recovery: Views from individuals with lived experience. *Journal of Clinical Psychology, 75*, 2119–2139.
18. Boone, S. D., & Brausch, A. M. (2016). Physical activity, exercise motivations, depression, and nonsuicidal self-injury in youth. *Suicide and Life-Threatening Behavior, 46*, 625–633.
19. Wallenstein, M. B., & Nock, M. K. (2007). Physical exercise as a treatment for non-suicidal self-injury: Evidence from a single case study. *American Journal of Psychiatry, 164*, 350–351.

20. Peterson, C., Ruch, W., Beermann, U., Park, N., & Seligman, M. E. P. (2007), Strengths of character, orientations to happiness, and life satisfaction. *Journal of Positive Psychology, 2*, 149–156.

21. Peterson, C., & Seligman, M. E. P. (2004). *Character strengths and virtues: A handbook and classification*. American Psychological Association; Oxford University Press.

22. Gillham, J., Adams-Deutsch, Z., Werner, J., Reivich, K., Coulter-Heindl, V., Linkins, M., Winder, B., Peterson, C., Park, N., Abenavoli, R., Contero, A., & Seligman, M. E. P. (2011). Character strengths predict subjective wellbeing during adolescence. *Journal of Positive Psychology, 6*, 31–44.

23. Park, N., Peterson, C., & Seligman, M. E. P. (2004). Strengths of character and well-being. *Journal of Social and Clinical Psychology, 23*, 603–619.

24. Kim, H. R., Kim, S. M., Hong, J. S., Han, D. H., Yoo, S., Min, K., & Lee, Y. S. (2018). Character strengths as protective factors against depression and suicidality among male and female employees. *BMC Public Health, 18*, 1084.

25. Zelkowitz, R. L., & Cole, D. A. (2019). Self-criticism as a transdiagnostic process in nonsuicidal self-injury and disordered eating: Systematic review and meta-analysis. *Suicide and Life-Threatening Behaviour, 49*, 310–327.

26. Jiang, Y., Ren, Y., Zhu, J., & You, J. (2020). Gratitude and hope relate to adolescent nonsuicidal self-injury: Mediation through self-compassion and family and school experiences. *Current Psychology, 41*, 935–942.

27. Ducasse, D., Dassa, D., Courtet, P., Brand-Apron, V., Walter, A., Guillaume, S., Jaussent, I., & Olié, E. (2019). Gratitude diary for the management of suicidal inpatients: A randomised controlled trial. *Depression and Anxiety, 36*, 400–411.

28. Southwell, S., & Gould, E. (2017). A randomised wait list-controlled pre-post-follow-up trial of a gratitude diary with a distressed sample. *Journal of Positive Psychology, 12*, 579–593.

29. Seligman, M. E. P., Steen, T. A., Park, N., & Peterson, C. (2005). Positive psychology progress: Empirical validation of interventions. *American Psychologist, 60*, 410–421.

30. Hooley, J. M., Fox, K. R., Wang, S. B., & Kwashie, A. N. D. (2018). Novel online daily diary interventions for nonsuicidal self-injury: A randomised controlled trial. *BMC Psychiatry, 18*, 264.

31. Seligman, M. E. (2012). *Flourish: A visionary new understanding of happiness and well-being*. Atria Paperback.

32. Bandel, S. L., & Brausch, A. M. (2020). Poor sleep associates with recent nonsuicidal self-injury engagement in adolescents. *Behavioural Sleep Medicine, 18*, 81–90.

33. Lan, Z., Huang, X., Zhou, H., & Chen, Z. (2020). Physical exercise, sleep quality and non-suicidal self-injury in adolescents: A meta-analysis review. *Revista Argentina de Clinica Psicológia, 29*, 1036–1047.

34. Liu, X., Chen, H., Bo, Q., Fan, F., & Jia, C. (2017). Poor sleep quality and nightmares are associated with non-suicidal self-injury in adolescents. *European Child and Adolescent Psychiatry, 26*, 271–279.

35. Schuch, F. B., Vancampfort, D., Richards, J., Rosenbaum, S., Ward, P. B., & Stubbs, B. (2016). Exercise as a treatment for depression: A meta-analysis adjusting for publication bias. *Journal of Psychiatric Research, 77*, 42–51.

36. Armey, M. F., Crowther, J. H., & Miller, I. W. (2011). Changes in ecological momentary assessment reported affect associated with episodes of nonsuicidal self-injury. *Behavior Therapy, 42*, 579–588.

37. Linehan, M. M. (2014). *DBT Skills training manual* (2nd ed). Guilford Press.

38. Campbell-Sills, L., Barlow, D. H., Brown, T. A., & Hoffmann, S. G. (2006). Effects of suppression and acceptance on emotional responses of individuals with anxiety and mood disorders. *Behaviour Research and Therapy, 44*, 1251–1263.

39. Gross, J. J., & Levenson, R. W. (1997). Hiding feelings: The acute effects of inhibiting negative and positive emotion. *Journal of Abnormal Psychology, 106*, 95–103.

40. Carver, C., Scheier, M., & Weintraub, J. (1989). Assessing coping strategies: A theoretically based approach. *Journal of Personality and Social Psychology, 52*, 267–283.

41. Stanley, B., & Brown, G. K. (2012). Safety planning intervention: A brief intervention to mitigate suicide risk. *Cognitive and Behavioural Practice, 19*, 256–264.

42. Lewis, S. P. (2016). The overlooked role of self-injury scars: Commentary and suggestions for clinical practice. *Journal of Nervous and Mental Disease, 204*, 33–35.

43. Lewis, S. P., & Hasking, P. (2021). Self-injury recovery: A person-centred framework. *Journal of Clinical Psychology, 77*, 884–895.

44. Burke, T. A., Ammerman, B. A., Hamilton, J. L., & Alloy, L. B. (2017). Impact of non-suicidal self-injury scale: Initial psychometric validation. *Cognitive Therapy and Research, 41*, 130–142.

45. Lewis, S. P., & Mehrabkhani, S. (2016). Every scar tells a story: Insight into people's self-injury scar experiences. *Counselling Psychology Quarterly, 29*, 296–310.

46. Burke, T. A., Piccirillo, M. L., Moore-Berg, S. L., Alloy, L. B., & Heimberg, R. G. (2019). The stigmatization of non-suicidal self-injury. *Journal of Clinical Psychology, 75*, 481–498.

47. Burke, T. A., Ammerman, B. A., Hamilton, J. L., Stange, J. P., & Piccirillo, M. (2020). Nonsuicidal self-injury scar concealment from the self and others. *Journal of Psychiatric Research, 130*, 313–320.

48. Staniland, L., Hasking, P., Boyes, M., & Lewis, S. (2021). Stigma and nonsuicidal self-injury: Application of a conceptual framework. *Stigma and Health, 6*(3), 312.

49. Hayes, S. C., Luoma, J. B., Bond, F. W., Masuda, A., & Lillis, J. (2006). Acceptance and commitment therapy: Model, processes and outcomes. *Behaviour Research and Therapy, 44*, 1–25.

50. Greene, K. (2009). An integrated model of health disclosure decision-making. In T. D. Afifi & W. A. Afifi (Eds.), *Uncertainty, information management, and disclosure decisions: Theories and applications* (pp. 226–253). Routledge/Taylor & Francis Group.

51. Chaudior, S., & Fisher, J. D. (2010). The disclosure process model: Understanding disclosure decision-making and post-disclosure outcomes among people living with a concealable stigmatized identity. *Psychological Bulletin, 136*, 236–256.

52. Kelada, L., Whitlock, J., Hasking, P., & Melvin, G. (2016). Parents' experiences of nonsuicidal self-injury among adolescents and young adults. *Journal of Child and Family Studies, 25*, 3403–3416.

53. Whitlock, J., Lloyd-Richardson, E., Fisseha, F., & Bates, T. (2018). Parental secondary stress: The often hidden consequences of nonsuicidal self-injury in youth. *Journal of Clinical Psychology, 74*, 178–196.

54. Rosenrot, S. A., & Lewis, S. P. (2020). Barriers and responses to the disclosure of non-suicidal self-injury: A thematic analysis. *Counselling Psychology Quarterly, 33*, 121–141.

55. Neff, K. (2003). Self-compassion: An alternative conceptualization of a healthy attitude toward oneself. *Self and Identity, 2*, 85–101.

56. Chio, F. H. N., Mak, W. W. S., & Yu, B. C. L. (2021). Meta-analytic review on the differential effects of self-compassion components on well-being and psychological distress: The moderating role of dialecticism on self-compassion. *Clinical Psychology Review, 85*, 101986.

57. Ferrari, M., Hunt, C., Harrysunker, A., Abbott, M. J., Beath, A. P., & Einstein, D. A. (2019). Self-compassion interventions and psychosocial outcomes: A meta-analysis of RCTs. *Mindfulness, 10*, 1455–1473.

Chapter 13

1. Lewis, S. P., & Hasking, P. A. (2021). Understanding self-injury: A person-centered approach. *Psychiatric Services, 72*(6), 721–723.

2. Lewis, S. P., & Hasking, P. (2019). Putting the "self" in self-injury research: Inclusion of people with lived experience in the research process. *Psychiatric Services, 70*(11), 1058–1060.

3. Rosenrot, S. A., & Lewis, S. P. (2020). Barriers and responses to the disclosure of non-suicidal self-injury: A thematic analysis. *Counselling Psychology Quarterly, 33*(2), 121–141.

4. Lewis, S. P., Bryant, L. A., Schaefer, B. M., & Grunberg, P. H. (2017). In their own words: Perspectives on nonsuicidal self-injury disorder among those with lived experience. *Journal of Nervous and Mental Disease, 205*(10), 771–779.

5. Lewis, S. P., & Hasking, P. A. (2021). Self-injury recovery: A person-centered framework. *Journal of Clinical Psychology, 77*(4), 884–895.

6. Klonsky, E. D., & Lewis, S. P. (2014). Assessment of non-suicidal self-injury. In M. K. Nock (Ed.), *Oxford handbook of suicide and self-injury* (pp. 337–354). Oxford University Press.

7. Walsh, B. (2007). Clinical assessment of self-injury: A practical guide. *Journal of Clinical Psychology, 63*(11), 1057–1068.

8. Walsh, B. W. (2012). *Treating self-injury: A practical guide*. Guilford Press.

9. Klonsky, E. D., Muehlenkamp, J., Lewis, S. P., & Walsh, B. (2011). *Nonsuicidal self-injury* (Vol. 22). Hogrefe Publishing.

10. Lewis, S. P., & Hasking, P. A. (2020). Rethinking self-injury recovery: A commentary and conceptual reframing. *BJPsych Bulletin, 44*(2), 44–46.

11. Lewis, S. P., Kenny, T. E., Whitfield, K., & Gomez, J. (2019). Understanding self-injury recovery: Views from individuals with lived experience. *Journal of Clinical Psychology, 75*(12), 2119–2139.

12. Gray, N., Hasking, P., & Boyes, M. E. (2021). The impact of ambivalence on recovery from non-suicidal self-injury: Considerations for health professionals. *Journal of Public Mental Health, 20*(4), 251–258.

13. Grunberg, P. H., & Lewis, S. P. (2015). Self-injury and readiness to recover: Preliminary examination of components of the stages of change model. *Counselling Psychology Quarterly, 28*(4), 361–371.

14. Hasking, P., Lewis, S. P., & Boyes, M. E. (2019). When language is maladaptive: Recommendations for discussing self-injury. *Journal of Public Mental Health, 18*(2), 148–152.

15. Hasking, P., & Boyes, M. (2018). Cutting words: A commentary on language and stigma in the context of nonsuicidal self-injury. *Journal of Nervous and Mental Disease, 206*(11), 829–833.

16. Hasking, P. A., Boyes, M. E., & Lewis, S. P. (2021). The language of self-injury: A data-informed commentary. *Journal of Nervous and Mental Disease, 209*(4), 233–236.

17. Lewis, S. P. (2017). I cut therefore I am? Avoiding labels in the context of self-injury. *Medical Humanities, 43*(3), 204.

18. Zelkowitz, R. L., & Cole, D. A. (2019). Self-criticism as a transdiagnostic process in nonsuicidal self-injury and disordered eating: Systematic review and meta-analysis. *Suicide and Life-Threatening Behavior, 49*(1), 310–327.

19. Burke, T. A., Hamilton, J. L., Cohen, J. N., Stange, J. P., & Alloy, L. B. (2016). Identifying a physical indicator of suicide risk: Non-suicidal self-injury scars predict suicidal ideation and suicide attempts. *Comprehensive Psychiatry, 65,* 79–87.

20. Burke, T. A., Olino, T. M., & Alloy, L. B. (2017). Initial psychometric validation of the non-suicidal self-injury scar cognition scale. *Journal of Psychopathology and Behavioral Assessment, 39*(3), 546–562.

21. Burke, T. A., Ammerman, B. A., Hamilton, J. L., Stange, J. P., & Piccirillo, M. (2020). Nonsuicidal self-injury scar concealment from the self and others. *Journal of Psychiatric Research, 130,* 313–320.

22. Lewis, S. P., & Mehrabkhani, S. (2016). Every scar tells a story: Insight into people's self-injury scar experiences. *Counselling Psychology Quarterly, 29*(3), 296–310.

23. Lewis, S. P. (2016). The overlooked role of self-injury scars: Commentary and suggestions for clinical practice. *Journal of Nervous and Mental Disease, 204*(1), 33–35.

Chapter 14

1. Lewis, S. P., & Hasking, P. (2020). Putting the self in self-injury research: Inclusion of people with lived experience in research. *Psychiatric Services, 70,* 1058–1060.

2. Lewis, S. P., & Hasking, P. (2021). Self-injury recovery: A person-centred framework. *Journal of Clinical Psychology, 77,* 884–895.

3. Victor, S. E., Lewis, S. P., & Muehlenkamp, J. J. (2022). Psychologists with lived experience of non-suicidal self-injury: Priorities, obstacles, and recommendations for inclusion. *Psychological Services, 19*(1), 21–28.

4. Lewis, S. P., Heath, N. L., & Whitley, R. (2022). Addressing self-injury stigma: The promise of innovative digital and video action-research methods. *Canadian Journal of Community Mental Health, 40*(3), 45–54.

5. Corrigan, P. W., & Watson, A. C. (2002). Understanding the impact of stigma on people with mental illness. *World Psychiatry, 1*(1), 16.

6. Corrigan, P. W., Watson, A. C., & Barr, L. (2006). The self–stigma of mental illness: Implications for self–esteem and self–efficacy. *Journal of Social and Clinical Psychology, 25*(8), 875–884.

7. Corrigan, P. W., Morris, S. B., Michaels, P. J., Rafacz, J. D., & Rüsch, N. (2012). Challenging the public stigma of mental illness: A meta-analysis of outcome studies. *Psychiatric Services, 63*(10), 963–973.

8. Thornicroft, G., Mehta, N., Clement, S., Evans-Lacko, S., Doherty, M., Rose, D., . . . Henderson, C. (2016). Evidence for effective interventions to reduce mental-health-related stigma and discrimination. *Lancet, 387*(10023), 1123–1132.

9. Jorm, A. F. (2020). Effect of contact-based interventions on stigma and discrimination: A critical examination of the evidence. *Psychiatric Services, 71*(7), 735–737.

10. Gibb, S. J., Beautrais, A. L., & Surgenor, L. J. (2010). Health-care staff attitudes towards self-harm patients. *Australian and New Zealand Journal of Psychiatry, 44*(8), 713–720.

11. Staniland, L., Hasking, P., Boyes, M., & Lewis, S. (2021). Stigma and nonsuicidal self-injury: Application of a conceptual framework. *Stigma and Health, 6*(3), 312.

12. Karman, P., Kool, N., Poslawsky, I. E., & van Meijel, B. (2015). Nurses' attitudes towards self-harm: A literature review. *Journal of Psychiatric and Mental Health Nursing, 22*(1), 65–75.

13. Saunders, K. E., Hawton, K., Fortune, S., & Farrell, S. (2012). Attitudes and knowledge of clinical staff regarding people who self-harm: A systematic review. *Journal of Affective Disorders, 139*(3), 205–216.

14. Berger, E., Hasking, P., & Reupert, A. (2014). Response and training needs of school staff towards student self-injury. *Teaching and Teacher Education, 44*, 25–34.

15. Heath, N. L., Toste, J. R., Sornberger, M. J., & Wagner, C. (2011). Teachers' perceptions of non-suicidal self-injury in the schools. *School Mental Health, 3*(1), 35–43.

16. Mitten, N., Preyde, M., Lewis, S., Vanderkooy, J., & Heintzman, J. (2016). The perceptions of adolescents who self-harm on stigma and care following inpatient psychiatric treatment. *Social Work in Mental Health, 14*(1), 1–21.

17. Rosenrot, S. A., & Lewis, S. P. (2020). Barriers and responses to the disclosure of non-suicidal self-injury: A thematic analysis. *Counselling Psychology Quarterly, 33*(2), 121–141.

18. Lloyd-Richardson, E. E., Lewis, S. P., Whitlock, J. L., Rodham, K., & Schatten, H. T. (2015). Research with adolescents who engage in non-suicidal self-injury: Ethical considerations and challenges. *Child and Adolescent Psychiatry and Mental Health, 9*(1), 1–14.

19. Muehlenkamp, J. J., Swenson, L. P., Batejan, K. L., & Jarvi, S. M. (2015). Emotional and behavioral effects of participating in an online study of nonsuicidal self-injury: An experimental analysis. *Clinical Psychological Science, 3*(1), 26–37.

20. Hasking, P., Rees, C. S., Martin, G., & Quigley, J. (2015). What happens when you tell someone you self-injure? The effects of disclosing NSSI to adults and peers. *BMC Public Health, 15*(1), 1–9.

21. Lewis, S. P., & Seko, Y. (2016). A double-edged sword: A review of benefits and risks of online nonsuicidal self-injury activities. *Journal of Clinical Psychology, 72*(3), 249–262.

22. Lewis, S. P., & Baker, T. G. (2011). The possible risks of self-injury web sites: A content analysis. *Archives of Suicide Research, 15*(4), 390–396.

23. Rodham, K., Gavin, J., Lewis, S. P., St. Denis, J. M., & Bandalli, P. (2013). An investigation of the motivations driving the online representation of self-injury: A thematic analysis. *Archives of Suicide Research, 17*(2), 173–183.

24. Lewis, S. P. (2017). I cut therefore I am? Avoiding labels in the context of self-injury. *Medical Humanities, 43*(3), 204.

25. Hasking, P., & Boyes, M. (2018). Cutting words: A commentary on language and stigma in the context of nonsuicidal self-injury. *Journal of Nervous and Mental Disease, 206*(11), 829–833.

26. Hasking, P., Lewis, S. P., & Boyes, M. E. (2019). When language is maladaptive: Recommendations for discussing self-injury. *Journal of Public Mental Health, 18*(2), 148–152.

27. Hasking, P. A., Boyes, M. E., & Lewis, S. P. (2021). The language of self-injury: A data-informed commentary. *Journal of Nervous and Mental Disease, 209*(4), 233–236.

28. Blades, C. A., Stritzke, W. G., Page, A. C., & Brown, J. D. (2018). The benefits and risks of asking research participants about suicide: A meta-analysis of the impact of exposure to suicide-related content. *Clinical Psychology Review, 64*, 1–12.

29. Corrigan, P. W., Kosyluk, K. A., & Rüsch, N. (2013). Reducing self-stigma by coming out proud. *American Journal of Public Health, 103*(5), 794–800.

30. Lewis, S. P., & Hasking, P. A. (2021). Understanding self-injury: A person-centered approach. *Psychiatric Services, 72*(6), 721–723.

31. Corrigan, P. W., & Kosyluk, K. A. (2013). Erasing the stigma: Where science meets advocacy. *Basic and Applied Social Psychology, 35*(1), 131–140.

32. Corrigan, P. W., Michaels, P. J., Vega, E., Gause, M., Larson, J., Krzyzanowski, R., & Botcheva, L. (2014). Key ingredients to contact-based stigma change: A cross-validation. *Psychiatric Rehabilitation Journal, 37*(1), 62.

33. American Psychiatric Association. (2013). *Diagnostic and Statistical Manual of Mental Disorders: Diagnostic and Statistical Manual of Mental Disorders* (5th ed.). American Psychiatric Association.

34. Favazza, A. R. (1998). The coming of age of self-mutilation. *Journal of Nervous and Mental Disease, 186*(5), 259–268.

35. Muehlenkamp, J. J. (2005). Self-injurious behavior as a separate clinical syndrome. *American Journal of Orthopsychiatry, 75*(2), 324–333.

36. Lengel, G. J., Ammerman, B. A., & Washburn, J. J. (2022). Clarifying the definition of nonsuicidal self-injury: Clinician and researcher perspectives. *Crisis: The Journal of Crisis Intervention and Suicide Prevention, 43*(2), 119–126.

37. Andover, M. S. (2014). Non-suicidal self-injury disorder in a community sample of adults. *Psychiatry Research, 219*(2), 305–310.

38. Muehlenkamp, J. J., Brausch, A. M., & Washburn, J. J. (2017). How much is enough? Examining frequency criteria for NSSI disorder in adolescent inpatients. *Journal of Consulting and Clinical Psychology, 85*, 611–619.

39. Washburn, J. J., Potthoff, L. M., Juzwin, K. R., & Styer, D. M. (2015). Assessing DSM-5 nonsuicidal self-injury disorder in a clinical sample. *Psychological Assessment, 27*, 31–41.

40. Ammerman, B. A., Lengel, G. J., & Washburn, J. J. (2021). Consideration of clinician and researcher opinions on the parameters of nonsuicidal self-injury disorder diagnostic criteria. *Psychiatry Research, 296*, 113642.

41. Lewis, S. P., Bryant, L. A., Schaefer, B. M., & Grunberg, P. H. (2017). In their own words: Perspectives on nonsuicidal self-injury disorder among those with lived experience. *Journal of Nervous and Mental Disease, 205*, 771–779.

42. Lewis, S. P., Kenny, T. E., Whitfield, K., & Gomez, J. (2019). Understanding self-injury recovery: Views from individuals with lived experience. *Journal of Clinical Psychology, 75*(12), 2119–2139.

43. Kelada, L., Hasking, P., Melvin, G., Whitlock, J., & Baetens, I. (2018). "I do want to stop, at least I think I do": An international comparison of recovery from nonsuicidal self-injury among young people. *Journal of Adolescent Research, 33,* 416–441.

44. Simone, A. C., & Hamza, C. A. (2020). Examining the disclosure of nonsuicidal self-injury to informal and formal sources: A review of the literature. *Clinical Psychology Review, 82,* 101907.

45. Park, Y., Mahdy, J. C., & Ammerman, B. A. (2021). How others respond to non-suicidal self-injury disclosure: A systematic review. *Journal of Community and Applied Psychology, 31,* 107–119.

46. Armiento, J. S., Hamza, C. A., & Willoughby, T. (2014). An examination of disclosure of nonsuicidal self-injury among university students. *Journal of Community and Applied Social Psychology, 24*(6), 518–533.

47. Burke, T. A., Piccirillo, M. L., Moore-Berg, S. L., Alloy, L. B., & Heimberg, R. G. (2019). The stigmatization of nonsuicidal self-injury. *Journal of Clinical Psychology, 75*(3), 481–498.

48. Lloyd, B., Blazely, A., & Phillips, L. (2018). Stigma towards individuals who self harm: Impact of gender and disclosure. *Journal of Public Mental Health, 17*(4), 184–194.

49. Devendorf, A. R. (2022). Is "me-search" a kiss of death in mental health research? *Psychological Services, 19*(1), 49–54.

50. Victor, S. E., Devendorf, A. R., Lewis, S. P., Rottenberg, J., Muehlenkamp, J. J., Stage, D. R. L., & Miller, R. H. (2022). Only human: mental-health difficulties among clinical, counseling, and school psychology faculty and trainees. *Perspectives on Psychological Science, 17*(6), 1576–1590.

51. Victor, S. E., Schleider, J. L., Ammerman, B. A., Bradford, D. E., Devendorf, A. R., Gruber, J., . . . Stage, D. R. L. (2022). Leveraging the strengths of psychologists with lived experience of psychopathology. *Perspectives on Psychological Science, 17*(6), 1624–1632.

52. Baum, F., MacDougall, C., & Smith, D. (2006). Participatory action research. *Journal of Epidemiology and Community Health, 60*(10), 854–857.

53. Cabassa, L. J., Nicasio, A., & Whitley, R. (2013). Picturing recovery: A photovoice exploration of recovery dimensions among people with serious mental illness. *Psychiatric Services, 64*(9), 837–842.

54. Gubrium, A., & Harper, K. (2016). *Participatory visual and digital methods* (Vol. 10). Routledge.

55. Ferrari, M., Rice, C., & McKenzie, K. (2015). ACE Pathways Project: Therapeutic catharsis in digital storytelling. *Psychiatric Services, 66*(5), 556.

56. Flanagan, E. H., Buck, T., Gamble, A., Hunter, C., Sewell, I., & Davidson, L. (2016). "Recovery speaks": A photovoice intervention to reduce stigma among primary care providers. *Psychiatric Services, 67*(5), 566–569.

57. Sitter, K. C. (2012). Participatory video: Toward a method, advocacy and voice (MAV) framework. *Intercultural Education, 23*(6), 541–554.

58. Buchanan, A., & Murray, M. (2012). Using participatory video to challenge the stigma of mental illness: A case study. *International Journal of Mental Health Promotion, 14*(1), 35–43.

59. Whitley, R., Sitter, K. C., Adamson, G., & Carmichael, V. (2021). A meaningful focus: Investigating the impact of involvement in a participatory video program on the recovery of participants with severe mental illness. *Psychiatric Rehabilitation Journal*, *44*(1), 63–69.

60. Bailey, D., Kemp, L., Wright, N., & Mutale, G. (2019). Talk about self-harm (TASH): Participatory action research with young people, GPs and practice nurses to explore how the experiences of young people who self-harm could be improved in GP surgeries. *Family Practice*, *36*(5), 621–626.

61. Ward, J., & Bailey, D. (2013). A participatory action research methodology in the management of self-harm in prison. *Journal of Mental Health*, *22*(4), 306–316.

62. Park, Y., Konge, L., & Artino, A. (2020). The positivism paradigm of research. *Academic Medicine*, *95*(5), 690–694.

63. Tolman, C. W. (Ed.). (1992). *Recent research in psychology: Positivism in psychology; Historical and contemporary problems.* Springer-Verlag Publishing.

64. Patton, M. Q. (2001). *Qualitative research and evaluation methods* (3rd ed.). Sage Publications.

65. Miller, E. (1999). Positivism and clinical psychology. *Clinical Psychology and Psychotherapy*, *6*(1), 1–6.

66. Breen, L. J., & Darlston-Jones, D. (2010). Moving beyond the enduring dominance of positivism in psychological research: Implications for psychology in Australia. *Australian Psychologist*, *45*(1), 67–76.

For the benefit of digital users, indexed terms that span two pages (e.g., 52–53) may, on occasion, appear on only one of those pages.

Tables, figures, and boxes are indicated by *t*, *f*, and *b* following the page number